PEDIATRIC QUICK REFERENCE

THIRD EDITION

Jeanette Garcia (handwritten signature)

Donna L. Wong, PhD, RN, PNP, CPN, FAAN

Adjunct Associate Professor
The University of Oklahoma
College of Medicine-Tulsa

Adjunct Professor
University of Oklahoma
College of Nursing

Adjunct Professor/Consultant
Oral Roberts University
Anna Vaughn School of Nursing
Tulsa, Oklahoma

Nursing Consultant
Children's Hospital at Saint Francis
Tulsa, Oklahoma
Texas Children's Hospital
Houston, Texas

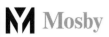

Mosby

An Affiliate of Elsevier Science

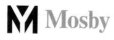

Mosby

An Affiliate of Elsevier Science

Editor-in-Chief: Sally Schrefer
Sr. Developmental Editor: Michele D. Hayden
Project Manager: Deborah L. Vogel
Production Editor: Ed Alderman
Cover Designer: Bill Drone

THIRD EDITION

Printed in the United States of America

Mosby, Inc.
An Imprint of Elsevier Science
11830 Westline Industrial Drive
St. Louis, Missouri 63146

ISBN 0-323-01056-3

03 KP / CG   9   8   7   6   5

CONTENTS

1 PHYSIOLOGIC ASSESSMENT, 1

Normal heart rates for infants and children, 1

Grading of pulses, 1

Electrode placement for standard chest I electrocardiograph monitoring, 2

Normal respiratory rates for children, 3

Classification of normal breath sounds, 3

Normal arterial blood gas and pH measurements, 4

Oxyhemoglobin dissociation curve, 5

Electrode placement for apnea monitoring, 6

Normal temperatures in children, 7

Temperature conversion formulas, 7

Temperature conversion chart, 7

Recommended bladder dimensions for blood pressure cuffs based on arm circumference, 8

Normative oscillometric (Dinamap) blood pressure values (systolic/diastolic; mean arterial pressure in parentheses), 8

Quick guide to blood pressure in children, 9

Definitions of blood pressure, 9

Normal blood pressure readings for boys, 10-11

Normal blood pressure readings for girls, 12-13

Pediatric coma scale, 14

2 PAIN ASSESSMENT AND MANAGEMENT, 15

Developmental characteristics of children's responses to pain, 15-16

Pain experience inventory, 17

CRIES neonatal postoperative pain scale, 18-20

FLACC scale, 21

Facial expression of physical distress in infant, 22

Wong-Baker FACES Pain Rating Scale, 23

Your child's pain rating scale, 24-25

Numeric scale for pain assessment, 26

Dosage recommendations for acetaminophen (Tylenol), 27

Dosage recommendations for ibuprofen (Children's Motrin), 28-30

Selected analgesics (equianalgesia), 31

Selected combination opioid and nonopioid oral analgesics—nonaspirin products, 32-33

Dosage of selected opioids for children, 34-35

Suggested medications for conscious sedation, 36

Routes and methods of analgesic drug administration, 37-43

Guidelines for converting from parenteral to oral analgesics, 44

Adverse effects of opioids, 44

Addiction vs tolerance and dependence, 45

Management of opioid-induced respiratory depression, 46

Guidelines for preventing withdrawal, 46

Guidelines for nonpharmacologic strategies for pain management, 47-51

3 FLUID REQUIREMENTS, 52

Ranges of daily water requirements at different ages under normal conditions, 52

Calculation of maintenance intravenous fluids for pediatric patients, 53

Assessment of urinary output, 53

4 INTRAMUSCULAR INJECTIONS, 54

Vastus lateralis site, 54

Ventrogluteal site, 55

Deltoid site, 56

Dorsogluteal site, 57

5   EMERGENCY INFORMATION, 58

Rapid cardiopulmonary assessment, 58
Guidelines for endotracheal tube and suction catheter sizes, 59
Cardiac arrest drugs, 60-61
First aid for choking, 62-63
Cardiopulmonary resuscitation (CPR), 64-65
Approximate weight per age, 66

6   COMMON LABORATORY TESTS, 67

7   RECOMMENDED SCHEDULE FOR IMMUNIZATION OF HEALTHY INFANTS AND CHILDREN, 84

8   SELECTED REFERENCES ON PAIN AND IMMUNIZATIONS, 85

NOTICE

For additional information on any topic in this book, the reader is referred to other books by Donna L. Wong, such as *Nursing Care of Infants and Children, Essentials of Pediatric Nursing,* and *Clinical Manual of Pediatric Nursing.*

1 PHYSIOLOGIC ASSESSMENT

NORMAL HEART RATES FOR INFANTS AND CHILDREN

Age	Beats/min	
	Resting (awake)	Resting (sleeping)
Newborn	100-180	80-160
1 wk to 3 mo	100-220	80-180
3 mo to 2 yr	80-150	70-120
2 to 10 yr	70-110	60-100
10 yr to adult	55-90	50-90

Modified from Gillette PC: Dysrhythmias. In Adams FH, Emmanouilides GC, Riemenschneider TA, editors: *Moss' heart disease in infants, children, and adolescents,* ed 4, Baltimore, 1989, Williams & Wilkins.

GRADING OF PULSES

Grade	Description
0	Not palpable
+1	Difficult to palpate, thready, weak, easily obliterated with pressure
+2	Difficult to palpate, may be obliterated with pressure
+3	Easy to palpate, not easily obliterated with pressure (normal)
+4	Strong, bounding, not obliterated with pressure

ELECTRODE PLACEMENT FOR STANDARD CHEST I ELECTROCARDIOGRAPHIC MONITORING

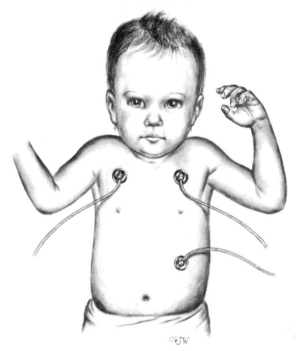

Electrodes with attached wires are often color coded:
- White for right
- Green (or red) for ground
- Black for left

NORMAL RESPIRATORY RATES FOR CHILDREN

Age	Rate (breaths/min)
Newborn	35
1-11 mo	30
2 yr	25
4 yr	23
6 yr	21
8 yr	20
10-12 yr	19
14-16 yr	17-18
18 yr	16-18

CLASSIFICATION OF NORMAL BREATH SOUNDS
Vesicular Breath Sounds
Heard over entire surface of lungs, with exception of upper
   intrascapular area and area beneath manubrium
Inspiration is louder, longer, and higher pitched than expiration
Sound is soft, swishing noise
Bronchovesicular Breath Sounds
Heard over manubrium and in upper intrascapular regions where
   trachea and bronchi bifurcate
Inspiration is louder and higher in pitch than in vesicular breathing
Bronchial Breath Sounds
Heard only over trachea near suprasternal notch
Inspiratory phase is short and expiratory phase is long

NORMAL ARTERIAL BLOOD GAS AND PH MEASUREMENTS*

pH: Normal range	**7.35-7.45**	
Acidosis	Mild:	7.30-7.35
	Moderate:	7.25-7.30
	Severe:	<7.25
Alkalosis	Mild:	7.45-7.50
	Moderate:	7.50-7.55
	Severe:	>7.55
P_{CO_2}: Normal range	**35-45 mm Hg**	
Hypercapnia	Mild:	45-50
	Moderate:	50-60
	Severe:	>60
Hypocapnia	Mild:	30-45
	Moderate:	25-30
	Severe:	<25
P_{O_2}: Normal range	**83-108 mm Hg**	
Hypoxemia	Mild:	55-85
	Moderate:	40-55
	Severe:	<40
Bicarbonate: Normal values	**21-28 mEq/liter**	
Depression	Mild:	19-22
	Moderate:	17-19
	Severe:	<17
Elevation	Mild:	28-31
	Moderate:	31-35
	Severe:	>35
Base excess: Normal values	**−3 to +3**	
Depression	Mild:	−3 to −7
	Moderate:	−7 through −10
	Severe:	<−10
Elevation	Mild:	+4 to +8
	Moderate:	+8 through +12
	Severe:	>+12

*Ranges are for children and infants beyond the newborn period.

OXYHEMOGLOBIN DISSOCIATION CURVE

Describes relationship between PaO_2 (arterial oxygen tension) and SaO_2 (arterial hemoglobin oxygen saturation).

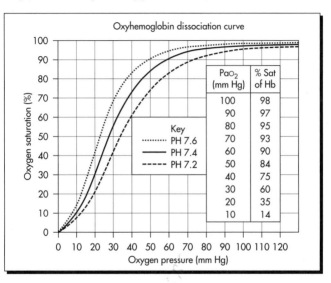

Changes in the affinity of hemoglobin for oxygen shift the position of the oxyhemoglobin dissociation curve.

Standard curve (middle curve above)—Assumes normal pH (7.4), temperature, PCO_2, and 2,3-DPG levels

Shift to left (upper curve above)—Increases O_2 affinity of Hb: increased pH; decreased temperature, PCO_2, and 2,3-DPG

Shift to right (lower curve above)—Decreases O_2 affinity of Hb: decreased pH; increased temperature, PCO_2, and 2,3-DPG

ELECTRODE PLACEMENT FOR APNEA MONITORING

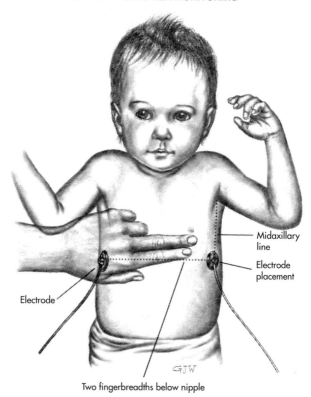

Midaxillary line

Electrode placement

Electrode

Two fingerbreadths below nipple

GJW

NOTE: In small infants, one fingerbreadth below nipple may be used.

NORMAL TEMPERATURES IN CHILDREN

Age	°F	Temperature	°C
3 mo	99.4		37.5
6 mo	99.5		37.5
1 yr	99.7		37.7
3 yr	99.0		37.2
5 yr	98.6		37.0
7 yr	98.3		36.8
9 yr	98.1		36.7
11 yr	98.0		36.7
13 yr	97.8		36.6

Modified from Lowrey GH: *Growth and development of children,* ed 8, St Louis, 1986, Mosby.

TEMPERATURE CONVERSION FORMULAS
$°F = (°C × ⅘) + 32$ or $(°C × 1.8) + 32$
$°C = (°F − 32) × ⅚$ or $(°F − 32) × 0.55$
$1° C = 1.8° F$

TEMPERATURE CONVERSION CHART
Selected Celsius to Fahrenheit Temperature Conversions

°C	°F	°C	°F	°C	°F
36.0	96.8	38.0	100.4	40.0	104.0
36.5	97.7	38.5	101.3	40.5	104.9
37.0	98.6	39.0	102.2	41.0	105.8
37.5	99.5	39.5	103.1	42.0	107.6

RECOMMENDED BLADDER DIMENSIONS FOR BLOOD PRESSURE CUFFS BASED ON ARM CIRCUMFERENCE

Arm circumference at midpoint (cm)	Cuff name*	Bladder width (cm)	Bladder length (cm)
5-7.5	Newborn	3	5
7.5-13	Infant	5	8
13-20	Child	8	13
24-32	Adult	13	24
32-42	Wide adult	17	32
42-50	Thigh	20	42

From Frohlich ED and others: Recommendations for human blood pressure determination by sphygmomanometers: report of a special task force appointed by the Steering Committee, American Health Association, *Circulation* 77:501A, 1988.

*Cuff name does not guarantee that the cuff will be appropriate size for a person within that age range.

NORMATIVE OSCILLOMETRIC (DINAMAP) BLOOD PRESSURE VALUES (SYSTOLIC/DIASTOLIC; MEAN ARTERIAL PRESSURE IN PARENTHESES)

Age	Mean	90th percentile	95th percentile
Newborn (1-3 days)	65/41 (50)	75/49 (59)	78/52 (62)
1 mo to 2 yr	95/58 (72)	106/68 (83)	110/71 (86)
2-5 yr	101/57 (74)	112/66 (82)	115/68 (85)

From Park M, Menard S: Normative oscillometric blood pressure values in the first 5 years in an office setting, *Am J Dis Child* 143(7):860-864, 1989.

QUICK GUIDE TO BLOOD PRESSURE IN CHILDREN

	Blood pressure (mm Hg)*	
Age	Systolic	Diastolic
2-6 mo	91	50 to 53
7-11 mo	90	47 + age in months
1-5 yr	90 + age in years	56
6-18 yr	83 + (2 × age in years)	52 + age in years

*Based on 50th percentile for males; slightly lower in females, especially 14 to 18 years of age.

DEFINITIONS OF BLOOD PRESSURE

Normal blood pressure—Systolic and diastolic pressures less than 90th percentile for age and sex

Normal high blood pressure—Systolic and diastolic pressures between the 90th and 95th percentiles for age and sex

Significant hypertension—Blood pressure persistently between 95th and 99th percentiles for age and sex

Severe hypertension—Blood pressure persistently at or above 99th percentile for age and sex

NORMAL BLOOD PRESSURE READINGS FOR BOYS

	Systolic blood pressure percentile			
Age	5th	50th	90th	95th
1 day	54	73	87	92
3 days	55	74	89	93
7 days	57	76	91	95
1 mo	67	86	101	105
2 mo	72	91	106	110
6 mo	72	90	105	109
1 yr	71	90	105	109
2 yr	72	91	106	110
3 yr	73	92	107	111
4 yr	74	93	108	112
5 yr	76	95	109	113
6 yr	77	96	111	115
7 yr	78	97	112	116
8 yr	80	99	114	118
9 yr	82	101	115	120
10 yr	84	102	117	121
11 yr	86	105	119	123
12 yr	88	107	121	126
13 yr	90	109	124	128
14 yr	93	112	126	131
15 yr	95	114	129	133
16 yr	98	117	131	136
17 yr	100	119	134	138
18 yr	102	121	136	140

Reprinted with permission from the Second Task Force on Blood Pressure Control in Children, National Heart, Lung and Blood Institute, Bethesda, MD. Tabular data prepared by Dr. B. Rosner, 1987.

| Age | Diastolic blood pressure* percentile | | | |
	5th	50th	90th	95th
1 day	38	55	68	72
3 days	38	55	68	71
7 days	37	54	67	71
1 mo	35	52	64	68
2 mo	33	50	63	66
6 mo	36	53	66	70
1 yr	39	56	69	73
2 yr	39	56	68	72
3 yr	39	55	68	72
4 yr	39	56	69	72
5 yr	40	56	69	73
6 yr	41	57	70	74
7 yr	42	58	71	75
8 yr	43	60	73	76
9 yr	44	61	74	78
10 yr	45	62	75	79
11 yr	47	63	76	80
12 yr	48	64	77	81
13 yr	45	63	77	81
14 yr	46	64	78	82
15 yr	47	65	79	83
16 yr	49	67	81	85
17 yr	51	69	83	87
18 yr	52	70	84	88

*Fourth Korotkoff sound (K4) was used for ages less than 13; K5 was used for ages 13 and over.

NORMAL BLOOD PRESSURE READINGS FOR GIRLS

Age	Systolic blood pressure percentile			
	5th	50th	90th	95th
1 day	46	65	80	84
3 days	53	72	86	90
7 days	60	78	93	97
1 mo	65	84	98	102
2 mo	68	87	101	106
6 mo	72	91	106	110
1 yr	72	91	105	110
2 yr	71	90	105	109
3 yr	72	91	106	110
4 yr	73	92	107	111
5 yr	75	94	109	113
6 yr	77	96	111	115
7 yr	78	97	112	116
8 yr	80	99	114	118
9 yr	81	100	115	119
10 yr	83	102	117	121
11 yr	86	105	119	123
12 yr	88	107	122	126
13 yr	90	109	124	128
14 yr	92	110	125	129
15 yr	93	111	126	130
16 yr	93	112	127	131
17 yr	93	112	127	131
18 yr	94	112	127	131

Reprinted with permission from the Second Task Force on Blood Pressure Control in Children, National Heart, Lung and Blood Institute, Bethesda, MD. Tabular data prepared by Dr. B. Rosner, 1987.

NORMAL BLOOD PRESSURE READINGS FOR GIRLS—cont'd

	Diastolic blood pressure* percentile			
Age	5th	50th	90th	95th
1 day	38	55	68	72
3 days	38	55	68	71
7 days	38	54	67	71
1 mo	35	52	65	69
2 mo	34	51	64	68
6 mo	36	53	66	69
1 yr	38	54	67	71
2 yr	40	56	69	73
3 yr	40	56	69	73
4 yr	40	56	69	73
5 yr	40	56	69	73
6 yr	40	57	70	74
7 yr	41	58	71	75
8 yr	43	59	72	76
9 yr	44	61	74	77
10 yr	46	62	75	79
11 yr	47	64	77	81
12 yr	49	66	78	82
13 yr	46	64	78	82
14 yr	49	67	81	85
15 yr	49	67	82	86
16 yr	49	67	81	85
17 yr	48	66	80	84
18 yr	48	66	80	84

*Fourth Korotkoff (K4) sound was used for ages less than 13; K5 was used for ages 13 and over.

PEDIATRIC COMA SCALE

NEUROLOGIC ASSESSMENT

Pupils	Right	Size		
		Reaction		
	Left	Size		
		Reaction		

++ = Brisk
+ = Sluggish
− = No reaction
C = Eye closed by swelling

Eyes open	Spontaneously	4	
	To speech	3	
	To pain	2	
	None	1	

Best motor response	Obeys commands	6	
	Localizes pain	5	
	Flexion withdrawal	4	
	Flexion abnormal	3	
	Extension	2	
	None	1	

Usually record best arm or age-appropriate response

Pupil scale (mm)

Best response to auditory and/or visual stimulus	>2 years		<2 years
	Orientation	5	5 Smiles, listens, follows
	Confused	4	4 Cries, consolable
	Inappropriate words	3	3 Inappropriate persistent cry
	Incomprehensible words	2	2 Agitated, restless
	None	1	1 No response
	Endotracheal tube or trach	T	
COMA SCALE TOTAL			

GLASGOW COMA SCALE

Pupil scale numbers: 1, 2, 3, 4, 5, 6, 7, 8

2 PAIN ASSESSMENT AND MANAGEMENT

DEVELOPMENTAL CHARACTERISTICS OF CHILDREN'S RESPONSES TO PAIN

Young Infants

Generalized body response of rigidity or thrashing, possibly with local reflex withdrawal of stimulated area

Loud crying

Facial expression of pain (brows lowered and drawn together, eyes tightly closed, mouth open and squarish; see p. 22)

Demonstrates no association between approaching stimulus and subsequent pain

Older Infants

Localized body response with deliberate withdrawal of stimulated area

Loud crying

Facial expression of pain and/or anger (same facial characteristics as pain but eyes may be open)

Physical resistance, especially pushing the stimulus away *after* it is applied

Young Children

Loud crying, screaming

Verbal expressions of "Ow," "Ouch," or "It hurts"

Thrashing of arms and legs

Continued

Attempts to push stimulus away *before* it is applied

Uncooperative; needs physical restraint

Requests termination of procedure

Clings to parent, nurse, or other significant person

Requests emotional support, such as hugs or other forms of physical comfort

May become restless and irritable with continuing pain

All these behaviors may be seen in anticipation of actual painful procedure.

School-Age Children

May see all behaviors of young child, especially *during* painful procedure but less in anticipatory period

Stalling behavior, such as "Wait a minute" or "I'm not ready"

Muscular rigidity, such as clenched fists, white knuckles, gritted teeth, contracted limbs, body stiffness, closed eyes, wrinkled forehead

Adolescents

Less vocal protest

Less motor activity

More verbal expressions, such as "It hurts" or "You're hurting me"

Increased muscle tension and body control

Data from Craig KD and others: Developmental changes in infant pain expression during immunization injections, *Soc Sci Med* 19(12):1331-1337, 1984; and Katz E, Kellerman J, Spiegel S: Behavioral distress in children with cancer undergoing medical procedures: developmental considerations, *J Consult Clin Psychol* 48(3):356-365, 1980.

PAIN EXPERIENCE INVENTORY
Questions for Parents

Describe any pain your child has had before.

How does your child usually react to pain?

Does your child tell you or others when he or she is hurting?

How do you know when your child is in pain?

What do you do to ease discomfort for your child when your child is hurting?

What does your child do to get relief from hurting?

Which of these actions work best to describe or take away your child's pain?

Is there anything special that you would like me to know about your child and pain? (If yes, have parents describe.)

Questions for Child

Tell me what pain is.

Tell me about the hurt you have had before.

What do you do when you hurt?

Do you tell others when you hurt?

What do you want others to do for you when you hurt?

What don't you want others to do for you when you hurt?

What helps the most to take away your hurt?

Is there anything special that you want me to know about you when you hurt? (If yes, have child describe.)

From Hester N, Barcus C: Assessment and management of pain in children. In *Pediatrics: nursing update* 1(14):3, Princeton, NJ, 1986, Continuing Professional Education Center.

CRIES NEONATAL POSTOPERATIVE PAIN SCALE

	0	1	2
Crying	No	High pitched	Inconsolable
Requires O_2 for Sat >95%	No	<30%	>30%
Increased vital signs	Heart rate and blood pressure = or < preoperative state	Heart rate and blood pressure increase <20% of preoperative state	Heart rate and blood pressure increase >20% of preoperative state
Expression	None	Grimace	Grimace/grunt
Sleepless	No	Wakes at frequent intervals	Constantly awake

Ages of use: 32-60 weeks gestational age. A score of 4 or higher indicates need for pain management.
Scoring range: 0 = no pain; 10 = worst pain.

CODING TIPS FOR USING CRIES

Crying	The characteristic cry of pain is *high pitched.* If no cry or cry that is not high pitched, **score 0.** If cry high pitched but infant is easily consoled, **score 1.** If cry is high pitched and infant is inconsolable, **score 2.**
Requires O_2 for Sat >95%	Look for *changes* in oxygenation. Infants experiencing pain manifest decreases in oxygenation as measured by Tco_2 or oxygen saturation. (Consider other causes of changes in oxygenation, such as atelectasis, pneumothorax, oversedation). If no oxygen is required, **score 0.** If <30% O_2 is required, **score 1.** If >30% is required, **score 2.**
Increased vital signs	Note: Measure blood pressure (BP) last, because this may wake child, causing difficulty with other assessments. Use baseline preoperative parameters from a nonstressed period.

Neonatal pain assessment tool developed at the University of Missouri–Columbia. Copyright S. Krechel, MD and J. Bildner, RNC, CNS, 1995. Used with permission. From Krechel SW, Bildner J: CRIES: a new neonatal postoperative pain measurement score: initial testing of validity and reliability. *Pediatr Anaesth* 5:53-61, 1995.

Continued

CODING TIPS FOR USING CRIES—cont'd

Increased vital signs—cont'd	Multiply baseline heart rate (HR) × 0.2, then add this to baseline HR to determine the HR that is 20% over baseline. Do likewise for BP. Use mean BP. If HR and BP are both unchanged or less than baseline, **score 0.** If HR or BP is increased but increase is <20% of baseline, **score 1.** If either one is increased >20% over baseline, **score 2.**
Expression	The facial expression most often associated with pain is a grimace. This may be characterized by lowered brow, eyes squeezed shut, deepening of the nasolabial furrow, and open lips and mouth. If no grimace is present, **score 0.** If grimace alone is present, **score 1.** If grimace and noncry vocalization grunt is present, **score 2.**
Sleepless	This parameter is scored based on the infant's state during the hour preceding this recorded score. If the child has been continuously asleep, **score 0.** If he/she has been awakened at frequent intervals, **score 1.** If he/she has been awake constantly, **score 2.**

FLACC SCALE

	0	1	2
Face	No particular expression or smile	Occasional grimace or frown, withdrawn, disinterested	Frequent to constant frown, clenched jaw, quivering chin
Legs	Normal position or relaxed	Uneasy, restless, tense	Kicking, or legs drawn up
Activity	Lying quietly, normal position, moves easily	Squirming, shifting back and forth, tense	Arched, rigid, or jerking
Cry	No cry (awake or asleep)	Moans or whimpers, occasional complaint	Crying steadily, screams or sobs, frequent complaints
Consolability	Content, relaxed	Reassured by occasional touching, hugging, or "talking to." Distractable	Difficult to console or comfort

Ages of use: 2 months to 7 years. *Scoring range:* 0 = no pain; 10 = worst pain.
From Merkel S, Voepel-Lewis T, Shayevitz J, Malviya S: The FLACC: a behavioral scale for scoring postoperative pain in young children, *Pediatr Nurs* 23(3):293-297, 1997. Used with permission of Jannetti Publications, Inc. and The University of Michigan Health System. Can be reproduced for clinical and research use.

FACIAL EXPRESSION OF PHYSICAL DISTRESS IN INFANT

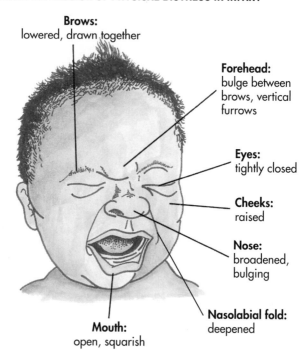

Brows: lowered, drawn together

Forehead: bulge between brows, vertical furrows

Eyes: tightly closed

Cheeks: raised

Nose: broadened, bulging

Nasolabial fold: deepened

Mouth: open, squarish

Facial expression of physical distress is the most consistent behavioral indicator of pain in infants.

May be reproduced for use in the clinical setting. From Wong DL: *Pediatric quick reference,* ed 3, St Louis, 2000, Mosby.

WONG-BAKER FACES PAIN RATING SCALE

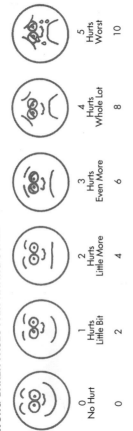

0 No Hurt	1 Hurts Little Bit	2 Hurts Little More	3 Hurts Even More	4 Hurts Whole Lot	5 Hurts Worst
0	2	4	6	8	10

Instructions: Point to each face using the words to describe the pain intensity. Ask the child to choose face that best describes own pain and record the appropriate number. *Rating scale is recommended for persons age 3 years and older.*

This tool may be reproduced for use in the clinical setting. From Wong DL: *Pediatric quick reference,* ed 3, St Louis, 2000, Mosby.

YOUR CHILD'S PAIN RATING SCALE*

Please keep a record of how well your child's pain medicines are working. Rate your child's pain before and after pain medicine is given.

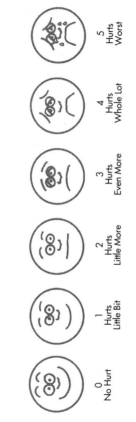

| 0 No Hurt | 1 Hurts Little Bit | 2 Hurts Little More | 3 Hurts Even More | 4 Hurts Whole Lot | 5 Hurts Worst |

Explain to your child that each face is for a person who has no hurt (pain) or some or a lot of hurt (pain). Point to each face and say the words under the face. Ask the child to pick the face that best describes how much hurt he (or she) has. Record the number of that face in the Pain Rating column. If your child's pain is above 2, or if you have other concerns with pain, let your nurse or physician know.

Date and time	Pain rating	Medicine the child took	Side effects, such as drowsiness or upset stomach

Pain assessment record. (Modified from Wong DL: Pain assessment in children. In Martin KS and others, editors: *Mosby's home health client teaching guides: Rx for teaching*, St Louis, 1997, Mosby.) May be photocopied for clinical use. From Wong DL: *Pediatric quick reference*, ed 3, St Louis, 2000, Mosby.

NUMERIC SCALE FOR PAIN ASSESSMENT

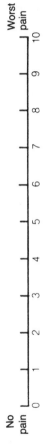

No pain | 0 1 2 3 4 5 6 7 8 9 10 | Worst pain

Explain to child that at one end of the line is a 0, which means that a person feels no pain (hurt). At the other end is a 10, which means the person feels the worst pain imaginable. The numbers 1 to 9 are for a very little pain to a whole lot of pain. Ask child to choose number that best describes own pain.

This tool may be reproduced for use in the clinical setting. From Wong DL: *Pediatric quick reference*, ed 3, St Louis, 2000, Mosby.

DOSAGE RECOMMENDATIONS FOR ACETAMINOPHEN (TYLENOL)*

Weight		Age		Infants' Concentrated Drops 80 mg/0.8 mL dropperful	Children's Suspension Liquid and Elixir 160 mg/5 mL teaspoon	Children's Chewable Tablets 80 mg each tablet	Junior Strength Chewable Tablets/Caplets 160 mg each tablet/caplet	Suppository† (not Tylenol) number/mg each suppository
Pounds	Kilos	Years						
6-11	2.7-5	0-3 mos		½				½ (80 mg)
12-17	5.4-7.7	4-11 mos		1	½			1 (80 mg)
18-23	8.2-10.4	12-23 mos		1½	¾			1 (120 mg)
24-35	10.9-15.9	2-3		2	1	2		1 (120 mg)
36-47	16.3-21.3	4-5			1½	3		2 (120 mg)
48-59	21.8-26.8	6-8			2	4		1 (325 mg)
60-71	27.2-32.2	9-10			2½	5	2	1 (325 mg)
72-95	32.7-43.1	11			3	6	2½	1½ (325 mg)
96	43.5	12					3	1½ (325 mg)
							4	2 (325 mg)

Modified from McNeil Consumer Products Company, Fort Washington, PA, 1997.

*Doses should be administered four or five times daily but should not exceed five doses or 75 mg/kg in 24 hours.

†Cut suppository in half *lengthwise*.

NOTE: Many other brands of acetaminophen are available, e.g., Panadol, Tempra, Liquiprin, Chewable Anacin 3, St. Joseph Aspirin Free Chewable, and Feverall suppositories.

May be reproduced for use in the clinical setting. From Wong DL: *Pediatric quick reference*, ed 3, St Louis, 2000, Mosby.

DOSAGE RECOMMENDATIONS FOR IBUPROFEN (CHILDREN'S MOTRIN)

Weight		Age	Chewable tablets 50 mg		
			Rx*		OTC*
			Fever under 39.2° C (102.5° F)	JRA†, pain, and fever ≥ 39.2° C (102.5° F)	
Pounds	Kilos	Years	5 mg/kg	10 mg/kg	7.5 mg/kg
12-17	5.4-7.7	6-11 mo			
18-23	8.2-10.4	12-23 mo	1 tab	2 tab	
24-35	10.9-15.9	2-3	1½ tab	3 tab	2 tab
36-47	16.3-21.3	4-5	2 tab	4 tab	3 tab
48-59	21.8-26.8	6-8	2½ tab	5 tab	
60-71	27.2-32.9	9-10	3 tab	6 tab	
72-95	32.7-43.1	11	4 tab	8 tab	

Modified from McNeil Consumer Products, Fort Washington, PA, June 1997. May be reproduced for use in the clinical setting. From Wong DL: *Pediatric quick reference,* ed 3, St Louis, 2000, Mosby.

DOSAGE RECOMMENDATIONS FOR IBUPROFEN (CHILDREN'S MOTRIN)—cont'd

Chewable tablets 100 mg			Caplets 100 mg		
Rx*		OTC*	Rx*		OTC*
Fever under 39.2° C (102.5° F)	JRA†, pain, and fever ≥ 39.2° C (102.5° F)		Fever under 39.2° C (102.5° F)	JRA,† pain, and fever ≥ 39.2° C (102.5° F)	
5 mg/kg	10 mg/kg	7.5 mg/kg	5 mg/kg	10 mg/kg	7.5 mg/kg
½ tab	1 tab				
¾ tab	1½ tab				
1 tab	2 tab		1 cap	2 cap	
1¼ tab	2½ tab	2 tab	1¼ cap	2½ cap	2 cap
1½ tab	3 tab	2½ tab	1½ cap	3 cap	2½ cap
2 tab	4 tab	3 tab	2 cap	4 cap	3 cap

Doses should be administered every 6 to 8 hours. Another form of nonprescription ibuprofen approved for children is Children's Advil.

*Rx indicates ibuprofen dose by prescription; OTC (over the counter) ibuprofen dose without a prescription.

†The recommended maximum daily dose for juvenile rheumatoid arthritis (JRA) is 30 to 40 mg/kg.   *Continued*

DOSAGE RECOMMENDATIONS FOR IBUPROFEN (CHILDREN'S MOTRIN)—cont'd

Weight		Age	Oral drops 50 mg/1.25 ml (1 dropperful)			Suspension 100 mg/5 ml		
			Rx*		OTC*	Rx		OTC*
			Fever under 39.2°C (102.5°F)	JRA†, pain, and fever ≥39.2°C (102.5°F)		Fever under 39.2°C (102.5°F)	JRA†, pain, and fever ≥39.2°C (102.5°F)	
Pounds	Kilos	Years	5 mg/kg	10 mg/kg	7.5 mg/kg	5 mg/kg	10 mg/kg	7.5 mg/kg
12-17	5.4-7.7	6-11 mo	½ dppr	1 dppr		¼ tsp	½ tsp	
18-23	8.2-10.4	12-23 mo	1 dppr	2 dppr		½ tsp	1 tsp	
24-35	10.9-15.9	2-3	1½ dppr	3 dppr	2 dppr	¾ tsp	1½ tsp	1 tsp
36-47	16.3-21.3	4-5				1 tsp	2 tsp	1½ tsp
48-59	21.8-26.8	6-8				1¼ tsp	2½ tsp	2 tsp
60-71	27.2-32.9	9-10				1½ tsp	3 tsp	2½ tsp
72-95	32.7-43.1	11				2 tsp	4 tsp	3 tsp

*Rx indicates ibuprofen dose by prescription; OTC (over the counter) ibuprofen dose without a prescription.
†The recommended maximum daily dose for juvenile rheumatoid arthritis (JRA) is 30 to 40 mg/kg.

SELECTED ANALGESICS (EQUIANALGESIA)

Drug	Equal to oral morphine (mg)	Equal to IM/IV morphine (mg)	Drug	Equal to oral morphine (mg)	Equal to IM/IV morphine (mg)
Hydromorphone (Dilaudid) 1 mg	4	1.3	Dolophine (Methadone) 10 mg	15.0	7.5
Codeine 30 mg	4.5	1.5	Acetaminophen (Tylenol) 325 mg	2.7	0.9
Meperidine (Demerol) 50 mg	4.8	1.6	Aspirin 325 mg	2.7	0.9
30 mg codeine + 300 mg acetaminophen (Tylenol No. 3)	7.2	2.4	Acetaminophen (Tylenol Extra Strength) 500 mg	4	1.3
Oxycodone 5 mg + 325 mg acetaminophen (Percocet)	7.2	2.4	60 mg codeine + acetaminophen 300 mg (Tylenol No. 4)	11.7	3.9
Oxycodone 5 mg + 325 mg aspirin (Percodan)	7.2	2.4	Transdermal fentanyl patch (Duragesic) (based on 25 µg/hr patch applied every 3 days = 50 mg oral morphine every 24 hr or divided into 6 doses = 8.3 mg)	8.3	2.77
Hydrocodone 5 mg + 500 mg acetaminophen (Vicodin, Lortab)	9	3			
Oxycodone 5 mg + 500 mg acetaminophen (Tylox)	9	3			

Courtesy of Betty R. Ferrell, PhD, FAAN, 1999. Used with permission.

*Oral medications with exception of Fentanyl.

SELECTED COMBINATION OPIOID AND NONOPIOID ORAL ANALGESICS–NONASPIRIN PRODUCTS*

Fioricet with Codeine	30 mg codeine
	325 mg acetaminophen
	50 mg butalbital
	40 mg caffeine
Hydrocet	5 mg hydrocodone
	500 mg acetaminophen
Lorcet-HD	5 mg hydrocodone
	500 mg acetaminophen
Lorcet Plus	7.5 mg hydrocodone
	650 mg acetaminophen
Lorcet 10/650	10 mg hydrocodone
	650 mg acetaminophen
Lortab 2.5/500	2.5 mg hydrocodone
	500 mg acetaminophen
Lortab 5/500	5 mg hydrocodone
	500 mg acetaminophen
Lortab 10/500	10 mg hydrocodone
	500 mg acetaminophen

---

*Aspirin is not recommended for children because of its possible association with Reye syndrome. Analgesic compounds with aspirin include Darvon Compound, Darvon with A.S.A., Percodan,† and Percodan-Demi.† Darvon or Darvocet (propoxyphene) is not recommended; its analgesic effect is no greater than that from aspirin, acetaminophen, or other NSAIDs. Propoxyphene, an opioid, can depress respirations. Its major metabolite is cardiotoxic and is a CNS simulant that can produce seizures. (Dahl JL: Darvon, a drug with dubious distinction, *Cancer Pain Update,* (48):3,6, Summer 1998.)

May be reproduced for use in the clinical setting. From Wong DL: *Pediatric quick reference,* ed 3, St Louis, 2000, Mosby.

Lortab Elixir (each 15 ml)	7.5 mg hydrocodone
	500 mg acetaminophen
Percocet-5†	5 mg oxycodone HCl
	325 mg acetaminophen
Tylenol with Codeine No. 1	7.5 mg codeine
	300 mg acetaminophen
Tylenol with Codeine No. 2	15 mg codeine
	300 mg acetaminophen
Tylenol with Codeine No. 3	30 mg codeine
	300 mg acetaminophen
Tylenol with Codeine No. 4	60 mg codeine
	300 mg acetaminophen
Tylenol and Codeine Elixir (each 5 ml)	12 mg codeine
	120 mg acetaminophen
	7% alcohol
Tylox†	5 mg oxycodone HCl
	500 mg acetaminophen
Vicodin	5 mg hydrocodone
	500 mg acetaminophen
Vicodin ES	7.5 mg hydrocodone
	750 mg acetaminophen
Vicodin HP	10 mg hydrocodone
	650 mg acetaminophen

---

†All medications require a prescription, but these are classified as schedule II drugs (like morphine), and each filling requires a written prescription that includes the patient's name and address, the practitioner's DEA (Drug Enforcement Agency) number, and the date. The prescription must be filled within 5 days.

DOSAGE OF SELECTED OPIOIDS FOR CHILDREN

Drug	Approximate equianalgesic oral dose	Approximate equianalgesic parenteral dose
Morphine[c]	30 mg every 3-4 hours (around-the-clock dosing)	10 mg every 3-4 hours
Fentanyl (Sublimaze) (oral mucosal form—Fentanyl Oralet)	1-1.5 mg	0.1 mg IV
Codeine[d]	200 mg every 3-4 hours	130 mg every 3-4 hours
Hydromorphone[c] (Dilaudid)	7.5 mg every 3-4 hours	1.5 mg every 3-4 hours
Hydrocodone (in Lorcet, Lortab, Vicodin, others)	30 mg every 3-4 hours	Not available
Levorphanol (Levo-Dromoran)	4 mg every 6-8 hours	2 mg every 6-8 hours
Meperidine (Demerol)[e]	300 mg every 2-3 hours	100 mg every 3 hours
Methadone (Dolophine, others)	20 mg every 6-8 hours	10 mg every 6-8 hours
Oxycodone (Roxicodone, Oxycontin; also in Percocet, Percodan, Tylox, others)	20-30 mg every 3-4 hours	Not available

Data from Acute Pain Management Guideline Panel: *Acute pain management: operative or medical procedures and trauma: clinical practice guideline:* AHCPR Pub No 92-0032, Rockville, MD, 1992, Agency for Health Care Policy and Research, Public Health Service, US Department of Health and Human Services; *Cancer pain relief and palliative care in children,* World Health Organization, Geneva, Switzerland, 1998; and Yaster M and others: *Pediatric pain management and sedation handbook,* St Louis, 1997, Mosby.

IV, Intravenous; *IM,* intramuscular; *PCA,* patient-controlled analgesia.

NOTE: Published tables vary in the suggested doses that are equianalgesic to morphine. Clinical response is the criterion that must be applied for each patient; titration to clinical response is necessary. Because there is not complete cross-tolerance among these drugs, it is usually necessary to use a lower than equianalgesic dose when changing drugs and to retitrate to response. Caution: Recommended doses do not apply to patients with renal or hepatic insufficiency or other conditions affecting drug metabolism and kinetics.

Recommended starting dose (children less than 50-kg body weight)[a]

Oral	Parenteral[b]
0.2-0.4 mg/kg every 3-4 hours	0.1-0.2 mg/kg IM every 3-4 hours
0.3-0.6 mg/kg time released every 12 hours	0.02-0.1 mg/kg IV bolus every 2 hours
	0.015 mg/kg every 8 minutes PCA
	0.01-0.02 mg/kg/hr IV infusion (neonates)
	0.01-0.06 mg/kg/hr IV infusion (child)
5-15 μg/kg; maximum dose 400 μg	0.5-1.5 μg/kg IV bolus every ½ hour
	1-2 μg/hr IV infusion
0.5-1 mg/kg every 3-4 hours	Not recommended
0.06 mg/kg every 3-4 hours	0.015 mg/kg IV bolus every 2-4 hours
0.2 mg/kg every 3-4 hours[f]	Not available
0.04 mg/kg every 6-8 hours	0.02 mg/kg every 6-8 hours
Not recommended	0.75 mg/kg every 2-3 hours
0.2 mg/kg every 6-8 hours	0.1 mg/kg every 6-8 hours
0.2 mg/kg every 3-4 hours[f]	Not available

[a]CAUTION: Doses listed for patients with body weight less than 50 kg should not be used as initial starting doses in infants less than 6 months of age. For nonventilated infants under 6 months of age, the initial opioid dose should be about one fourth to one third of the dose recommended for older infants and children. For children with body weight greater than 50 kg, the usual adult dose should be used.

[b]IM injections should not be used.

[c]For morphine, hydromorphone, and oxymorphone, rectal administration is an alternate route for patients unable to take oral medications, but equianalgesic doses may differ from oral and parenteral doses because of pharmacokinetic differences.

[d]CAUTION: Codeine doses above 65 mg often are not appropriate because of diminishing incremental analgesia with increasing doses but continually increasing constipation and other side effects.

[e]Meperidine is not recommended for continuous pain control (i.e., postoperatively) because of risk of normeperidine toxicity.

[f]CAUTION: Doses of aspirin and acetaminophen in combination with opioid/NSAID preparations must also be adjusted to patient's body weight.

SUGGESTED MEDICATIONS FOR CONSCIOUS SEDATION
*OPIOIDS**

Morphine sulfate, 0.05 to 0.10 mg/kg IV over 1 to 2 minutes given 5 minutes before procedure

Fentanyl, 1 to 2 µg/kg (0.001 to 0.002 mg/kg) IV 3 minutes before procedure

Fentanyl Oralet, 5 to 15 µg/kg, maximum to 400 µg, orally 20 to 40 minutes before procedure†

Hydromorphone (Dilaudid), 0.015-0.02 mg/kg IV over 1 to 2 minutes given 5 minutes before procedure.

Meperidine (if morphine sulfate or fentanyl is not available), 0.5 to 1.0 mg/kg IV over 1 to 2 minutes given 2 to 5 minutes before procedure or 1.5 mg/kg orally 45 to 60 minutes before procedure

---

Modified from Zeltzer LK and others: Report of the subcommittee on the management of pain associated with procedures in children with cancer, *Pediatrics* 86(suppl):826-831, 1990; Coté CJ: Sedation for the pediatric patient, *Pediatr Clin North Am* 41(1):31-58, 1994; and Yaster M, and others: *Pediatric pain management and sedation handbook,* St Louis, 1997, Mosby.
*Provide analgesia and sedation.

†Not recommended for children less than 15 kg. Lozenge should be sucked, not chewed and swallowed. If chewed, drug is less effective because part of it is metabolized by liver before entering bloodstream. Swallowing drug rapidly does not increase risk of respiratory depression during first 15 to 30 minutes, period of greatest risk for decreased respiration.

May be reproduced for use in the clinical setting. From Wong DL: *Pediatric quick reference,* ed 3, St Louis, 2000, Mosby.

SEDATIVES*

Midazolam (Versed), 0.25 to 0.5 mg/kg (children 6 months to less than 6 years of age and less cooperative children may require a higher dose of up to 1 mg/kg), maximum to 20 mg, using oral preparation, 10 to 20 minutes, or 0.05 mg/kg IV 3 minutes before procedure

Diazepam (Valium), 0.2 to 0.3 mg/kg, maximum to 10 mg, orally 45 to 60 minutes before procedure

Pentobarbital (Nembutal), 1 to 3 mg/kg IV boluses to maximum of 100 mg until asleep

Chloral hydrate, 50 to 75 mg/kg, to maximum of 100 mg/kg or 2.5 g, orally or rectally 60 minutes before procedure

ROUTES AND METHODS OF ANALGESIC DRUG ADMINISTRATION
ORAL

Preferred because of convenience, cost, and relatively steady blood levels

Higher dosages of oral form of opioids required for equivalent parenteral analgesia

Peak drug effect occurs after 1½ to 2 hours for most analgesics
> Delay in onset is disadvantage when rapid control of severe pain or fluctuating pain is desired

SUBLINGUAL/BUCCAL/TRANSMUCOSAL

Tablet or liquid placed between cheek and gum (buccal) or under tongue (sublingual)

Highly desirable because more rapid onset than oral
> Less first-pass effect through liver than oral route which normally reduces analgesia from oral opioids (unless sublingual/buccal form swallowed, which occurs often in children)

---

*Provide sedation but no analgesia.

Few drugs commercially available in this form

Many drugs can be compounded into a sublingual troche or lozenge*

Fentanyl Oralet—oral transmucosal fentanyl citrate in hard confection base on a plastic holder used for preoperative or preprocedural sedation/analgesia

Actiq—same formulation as Fentanyl Oralet; indicated only for management of breakthrough cancer pain in patients with malignancies who are already receiving and who are tolerant to opioid therapy.

INTRAVENOUS (IV) (BOLUS)

Preferred for rapid control of severe pain

Provides most rapid onset of effect, usually in about 5 minutes

Advantage for acute pain, procedural pain, and "breakthrough" pain

Initial bolus dose is controversial; one recommendation is one-half IM dose

Needs to be repeated hourly for continuous pain control

Drugs with short half-life (morphine, fentanyl, hydromorphone) are preferred, to avoid toxic accumulation of drug

INTRAVENOUS (CONTINUOUS)

Preferred over bolus and IM for maintaining control of pain

Provides steady blood levels

Data primarily from American Pain Society: *Principles of analgesic use in the treatment of acute pain or cancer pain,* ed 4, Glenview, IL, 1999, The Society; and McCaffery M, Pasero C: *Pain: clinical manual,* ed 2, St Louis, 1999, Mosby. *For further information about compounding drugs in troches or suppositories, contact Technical Staff, Professional Compounding Centers of America, Houston, TX: (800) 331-2498, Web site: www.thecompounders.com.

Easy to titrate dosage

Amount of initial dose is controversial; one approach to calculating hourly infusion rate is to divide IM dose by drug's expected duration for IM route

Peak effect is delayed; for rapid pain relief, begin with initial IV bolus dose (see above)

SUBCUTANEOUS (SC) (CONTINUOUS)

Used when oral and IV routes not available

Provides equivalent blood levels to continuous IV infusion

Suggested initial bolus dose to equal 2-hour IV dose; total 24-hour dose usually equal to total IV or IM 24-hour dose

PATIENT-CONTROLLED ANALGESIA (PCA)

Generally refers to self-administration of drugs, regardless of route

Typically uses programmable infusion pump (IV, epidural, or SC) that permits self-administration of boluses of medication at preset dose and time interval (*lockout interval* is time between doses)

"PCA" bolus administration may be combined with initial bolus and continuous (basal or background) infusion of opioid

Suggested Intravenous Patient Controlled Analgesia Opioid Infusion Orders

Drug	Basal rate µg/kg/hr	Bolus rate µg/kg/dose	Lockout period minutes	Maximum dose/hour mg/kg
Morphine	10-30	10-30	6-10	0.1-0.15
Hydromorphone	3-5	3-5	6-10	0.015-0.02
Fentanyl	0.5-1.0	0.5-1.0	6-10	0.002-0.004

From Yaster M, Krane EJ, Kaplan RF, et al: *Pediatric pain management and sedation handbook,* St Louis, 1997, Mosby. Used with permission.

Optimum lockout interval not known, but must be at least as long as time needed for onset of drug

Should effectively control pain during movement or procedures

Longer lockout requires larger dose

INTRAMUSCULAR (IM)

NOT RECOMMENDED FOR PAIN CONTROL

Painful administration (hated by children)

Some drugs (e.g., meperidine) can cause tissue damage

Wide fluctuation in absorption of drug from muscle

INTRADERMAL

Used primarily for skin anesthesia (e.g., for lumbar puncture, bone marrow aspiration, venous and arterial puncture, skin biopsy)

Local anesthetics (lidocaine) cause stinging, burning sensation

Duration of stinging may depend on type of "caine" used

To avoid stinging sensation associated with lidocaine:

Buffer the solution by addition 1 part sodium bicarbonate (1 mEq/ml) to 10 parts 1% or 2% lidocaine

Change needle used to withdraw BL to 30-gauge needle for intradermal injection

For venipuncture or port access, inject 0.1 ml or less BL intradermally directly over intended puncture site; anesthesia occurs almost immediately

Suggested maximum dose of lidocaine for local anesthesia is 4.5 mg/kg

If buffering lidocaine vial (e.g., 20 ml lidocaine with 2 ml sodium bicarbonate), solution may be used for 7 days if unrefrigerated or 14 days if refrigerated

---

Data primarily from American Pain Society: *Principles of analgesic use in the treatment of acute pain or cancer pain,* ed 4, Glenview, IL, 1999, The Society; and McCaffery M, Pasero C: *Pain: clinical manual,* St Louis, ed. 2, 1999, Mosby.

TOPICAL/TRANSDERMAL

EMLA (Eutectic Mixture of Local Anesthetics
[lidocaine/prilocaine]) cream and Anesthetic Disc

Eliminates or reduces pain from most procedures involving skin puncture

Must be placed over puncture site under occlusive dressing or as Anesthetic Disc for 1 hour or more before procedure

LAT (Lidocaine/Adrenaline/Tetracaine)
or Tetracaine/Phenylephrine (Tetraphen)

Provides skin anesthesia about 15 minutes after application

GEL (preferably) or liquid placed on wounds for suturing (nonintact skin)

Cocaine should no longer be used because of the risk of systemic absorption and toxicity

Adrenalin must not be used on end arterioles (fingers, toes, tip of nose, penis, earlobes) because of vasoconstriction

Numby Stuff

Uses iontophoresis to transport lidocaine 2% and epinephrine 1:100,000 *(Iontocaine)* into the skin

A small battery-powered electronic device delivers electric current via an electrode with Iontocaine and a ground electrode

Produces local dermal anesthesia in about 10 minutes to a depth of approximately 10 mm at maximum setting

May be frightening to young children when they see the device and feel the mild current

Child should be observed during iontophoresis

Transdermal Fentanyl (Duragesic)

Available as "patch" for continuous cancer pain control

Safety and efficacy not established in children under 12 years

Not appropriate for initial relief of acute pain because of long interval to peak effect (from 12 to 24 hours); for rapid onset of pain relief, an immediate release opioid must be given

Orders for "rescue doses" of an immediate release opioid should be available for ***breakthrough pain,*** a flare of severe pain that "breaks through" the medication that is being administered at regular intervals for persistent pain.

Has duration of up to 72 hours for prolonged pain relief

If respiratory depression occurs, several doses of naloxone may be needed

Vapocoolant

Use of spray coolant, such as Fluori-Methane, Frigiderm, or ethyl chloride, immediately placed on the skin before the needle puncture

Some children dislike the cold; spraying the coolant on a cotton ball first and then on the skin may be less uncomfortable

Application of ice to the skin for 30 seconds was found to be ineffective

RECTAL

Alternative to oral or parenteral routes

Variable absorption rate

Generally disliked by children

Many drugs can be compounded into rectal suppositories*

---

*For further information about compounding drugs in troches or suppositories, contact Technical Staff, Professional Compounding Centers of America, Houston, TX, (800) 331-2498, Web site: www.thecompounders.com.

REGIONAL NERVE BLOCK

Use of long-acting anesthetic (bupivacaine or ropivacaine) injected into nerves to block pain at site

Provides prolonged analgesia postoperatively, such as after inguinal herniorrhaphy

May be used to provide local anesthesia for surgery, such as dorsal penile nerve block for circumcision, or for reduction of fractures

INHALATION

Use of anesthetics, such as nitrous oxide or halothane, to produce partial or complete analgesia for painful procedures

Occupational exposure to high levels of nitrous oxide may cause side effects

EPIDURAL/INTRATHECAL

Involves catheter placed into epidural, caudal, or intrathecal space for continuous infusion or single or intermittent administration of opioid (with or without a long-acting anesthetic, e.g., bupivacaine or ropivacaine)

Analgesia primarily from drug's direct effect on opioid receptors in spinal cord

Respiratory depression is rare but may have slow and delayed onset; can be prevented by checking level of sedation and respiratory rate and depth hourly for initial 24 hours and decreasing dose when excessive sedation is detected

Nausea, itching, and urinary retention are common dose-related side effects from the epidural opioid

Mild hypotension, urinary retention, and temporary motor and/or sensory deficits are common unwanted effects of epidural local anesthetic

GUIDELINES FOR CONVERTING FROM PARENTERAL TO ORAL ANALGESICS

Convert directly by giving next dose of analgesic orally (PO) in equivalent dosage without any parenteral form of the same drug.

or

Convert gradually to PO form using the following steps:

Convert half the parenteral dose to a PO dose.

Administer half the parenteral dose and the PO dose.

Assess pain relief.

If pain relief is inadequate, increase the PO dose as needed.

If sedation occurs, decrease the PO dose as needed.

When the parenteral and PO doses are effective, discontinue the parenteral dose and give twice the PO dose.

ADVERSE EFFECTS OF OPIOIDS
General Side Effects

Respiratory depression

Sedation

Constipation (possibly severe)

Nausea and vomiting

Agitation, euphoria

Mental clouding

Hallucinations

Orthostatic hypotension

Pruritus

Urticaria

Sweating

Miosis

Anaphylaxis (rare)

Signs of Tolerance

Decreasing pain relief

Decreasing duration of pain relief

Signs of Withdrawal from Physical Dependence

Initial Signs of Withdrawal

Lacrimation

Rhinorrhea

Yawning

Sweating

Later Signs of Withdrawal

Restlessness, irritability

Tremors

Anorexia

Dilated pupils

Gooseflesh

ADDICTION VS TOLERANCE AND DEPENDENCE

Signs of tolerance and physical dependence must not be confused with addiction. These terms reflect completely different behavioral and physiologic actions:

Physical dependence on an opioid is a physiologic state in which abrupt cessation of the opioid, or administration of an opioid antagonist, results in a withdrawal syndrome. It is an expected occurrence in all individuals in the presence of continuous use of opioids for therapeutic or for nontherapeutic purposes. It does not, in and of itself, imply addiction.

Tolerance is a form of neuroadaptation to the effects of chronically administered opioids (or other medications). It is indicated by the need for increasing or more frequent doses of the medication to achieve the initial effects of the drug. Tolerance may occur both to the analgesic effects of opioids and to some of the unwanted side effects, such as respiratory depression, sedation, and nausea. The occurrence of tolerance is variable in occurrence but does not, in and of itself, imply addiction.

Addiction in the context of pain treatment with opioids is characterized by a persistent pattern of dysfunctional opioid use that may involve any or all of the following: adverse consequences associated with the use of opioids; loss of control over the use of opioids; and preoccupation with obtaining opioids, despite the presence of adequate analgesia.

Individuals who have severe, unrelieved pain may become intensely focused on finding relief for their pain. Sometimes such patients may appear to be preoccupied with obtaining opioids, but the preoccupation is with finding relief of pain, rather than using opioids. This phenomenon has been termed ***pseudoaddiction.***

From American Society of Addiction Medicine: *Public policy statement on the rights and responsibilities of physicians in the use of opioids for the treatment of pain,* April 16, 1997.

MANAGEMENT OF OPIOID-INDUCED RESPIRATORY DEPRESSION

1. Stop or reduce infusion by 25% when possible
2. Stimulate patient (shake gently, call by name, ask to breathe)
3. Administer oxygen (consider naloxone [Narcan])
4. If patient cannot be aroused or is apneic, administer naloxone*
   - For children less than 40 kg: dilute 0.1 mg of naloxone in 10 ml of sterile saline to make 10 μg/ml solution and give 0.5 μg/kg
   - For children over 40 kg: dilute 0.4 mg ampule in 10 ml of sterile saline and give 0.5 ml
   - Administer bolus IV push every 2 minutes until effect is obtained
5. Closely monitor patient. Naloxone's duration of antagonist action may be shorter than that of opioid, requiring repeated doses of naloxone, and naloxone can precipitate withdrawal.

NOTE: Flumazenil (Romazicon) reverses benzodiazepine-induced respiratory depression, e.g., midazolam (Versed). Pediatric dosing experience suggest 0.01 mg/kg (0.1 ml/kg) as initial dose; if inadequate or no response within 1-2 minutes, administer same dose and repeat as needed at 1-minute intervals until maximum dose of 1 mg (10 ml).

GUIDELINES FOR PREVENTING WITHDRAWAL*

1. Gradually reduce dose (similar to tapering of steroids):
   Give one half of previous daily dose every 6 hours for first 2 days
   Then reduce dose by 25% every 2 days
2. Continue this schedule until total daily dose of 0.6 mg/kg/day of morphine (or equivalent) is reached
3. After 2 days on this dose, discontinue opioid

---

*American Pain Society: *Principles of analgesic use in the trreatment of acute pain and cancer pain,* ed. 4, Glenview, IL, 1999, The Society.

4. May also switch to oral methadone, using one fourth of equianalgesic dose as initial weaning dose and proceeding as just described

GUIDELINES FOR NONPHARMACOLOGIC STRATEGIES FOR PAIN MANAGEMENT
General Strategies

Use nonpharmacologic interventions to supplement, not replace, pharmacologic interventions; use for mild pain and pain that is reasonably well controlled with analgesics.

Form a trusting relationship with child and family.

Express concern regarding their reports of pain and intervene appropriately.

Take an active role in seeking effective pain management strategies.

Use general guidelines to prepare child for procedure

Prepare child before potentially painful procedures but avoid "planting" the idea of pain. For example, instead of saying, "This is going to (or may) hurt," say, "Sometimes this feels like pushing, sticking, or pinching, and sometimes it doesn't bother people. Tell me what it feels like to you."

Use "nonpain" descriptors when possible (e.g., "It feels like heat" rather than "It's a burning pain").

This allows for variation in sensory perception, avoids suggesting pain, and gives child control in describing reactions.

Avoid evaluative statements or descriptions (e.g., "This is a terrible procedure" or "It really will hurt a lot").

Stay with child during a painful procedure.

Allow parents to stay with child if child and parent desire; encourage parent to talk softly to child and to remain near child's head.

Involve parents in learning specific nonpharmacologic strategies and assisting child in their use. *Continued*

Educate child about the pain, especially when explanation may lessen anxiety (e.g., that pain may occur after surgery and does not indicate something is wrong; reassure that child is not responsible for the pain).

For long-term pain control, give child a doll, which becomes "the patient," and allow child to do everything to the doll that is done to the child; pain control can be emphasized through the doll by stating, "Dolly feels better after the medicine."

Teach procedures to child and family for later use.

Specific Strategies

Distraction

Involve parent and child in identifying strong distractors.

Involve child in play; use radio, tape recorder, CD player; have child sing or use rhythmic breathing.

Have child take a deep breath and blow it out until told to stop.*

Have child blow bubbles to "blow the hurt away."

Have child concentrate on yelling or saying "ouch" by focusing on "yelling loud or soft as you feel it hurt: that way I know what's happening."

Have child look through kaleidoscope (type with glitter suspended in fluid-filled tube) and encourage to concentrate by asking, "Do you see the different designs?"†

Use humor, such as watching cartoons, telling jokes or funny stories, or acting silly with child.

Have child read, play games, or visit with friends.

---

*French GM, Painter EC, Courty DL. Blowing away shot pain: a technique for pain management during immunization, *Pediatrics* 93(3):384-388, 1994.

†Vessey JA, Carlson KL, McGill J: Use of distraction with children during an acute pain experience, *Nurs Res* 43(6):369-372, 1994.

Relaxation

With an infant or young child:

Hold in a comfortable, well-supported position, such as vertically against the chest and shoulder.

Rock in a wide, rhythmic arc in a rocking chair or sway back and forth, rather than bouncing child.

Repeat one or two words softly, such as "Mommy's here."

With a slightly older child:

Ask child to take a deep breath and "go limp as a rag doll" while exhaling slowly, then ask child to yawn (demonstrate if needed).

Help child assume a comfortable position (e.g., pillow under neck and knees)

Begin progressive relaxation: starting with the toes, systematically instruct child to let each body part "go limp" or "feel heavy"; if child has difficulty with relaxing, instruct child to tense or tighten each body part and then relax it.

Allow child to keep eyes open, since children may respond better if eyes are open rather than closed during relaxation.

Guided Imagery

Have child identify some highly pleasurable real or pretend experience.

Have child describe details of the event, including as many senses as possible (e.g., "feel the cool breezes," "see the beautiful colors," "hear the pleasant music").

Have child write down or tape record script.

Encourage child to concentrate only on the pleasurable event during the painful time; enhance the image by recalling specific details, such as reading the script or playing the tape.

Combine with relaxation and rhythmic breathing.

Continued

Positive Self-Talk

Teach child positive statements to say when in pain (e.g., "I will be feeling better soon," "When I go home, I will feel better, and we will eat ice cream.")

Thought Stopping

Identify positive facts about the painful event (e.g., "It does not last long").

Identify reassuring information (e.g., "If I think about something else, it does not hurt as much").

Condense positive and reassuring facts into a set of brief statements, and have child memorize them (e.g., "Short procedure, good veins, little hurt, nice nurse, go home").

Have child repeat the memorized statements whenever thinking about or experiencing the painful event.

Cutaneous Stimulation

Includes simple rhythmic rubbing; use of pressure, electric vibrator; massage with hand lotion, powder, or menthol cream; application of heat or cold, such as vapocoolant spray on the site before giving injection or application of ice to the site opposite the painful area (e.g., if right knee hurts, place ice on left knee).

A more sophisticated method is **transcutaneous electrical nerve stimulation (TENS)** (use of controlled low-voltage electricity to the body via electrodes placed on the skin).

Another method is the use of **therapeutic electro membrane (TEM),** a high technology membrane electron reservoir fabricated from a non-woven, nonallergenic dressing that, when placed in contact with the skin, releases the stored electrons in the form of micro-current impulses.*

Behavioral Contracting

Informal—May be used with children as young as 4 or 5 years of age:
   Use stars or tokens as rewards.
   Give uncooperative or procrastinating children (during a procedure) a limited time (measured by a visible timer) to complete the procedure.
   Proceed as needed if child is unable to comply.
   Reinforce cooperation with a reward if the procedure is accomplished within specified time.

Formal—Use written contract, which includes the following:
   Realistic (seems possible) goal or desired behavior
   Measurable behavior (e.g., agrees not to hit anyone during procedures)
   Contract written, dated, and signed by all persons involved in any of the agreements
   Identified rewards or consequences are reinforcing.
   Goals can be evaluated
   Requires commitment and compromise from both parties (e.g., while timer is used, nurse will not nag or prod child to complete procedure).

---

*For more information contact Helio Medical Supplies, Inc., 2080A Walsh Avenue, Santa Clara, CA 95050; (888)-PAINTEM (888-724-6836); e-mail: eileen@heliomed.com

3 FLUID REQUIREMENTS

RANGES OF DAILY WATER REQUIREMENTS AT DIFFERENT AGES UNDER NORMAL CONDITIONS

Age	Total water requirements per 24 hr (ml)	Water requirements per kg per 24 hr (ml)
3 days	250-300	80-100
10 days	400-500	125-150
3 mo	750-850	140-160
6 mo	950-1100	130-155
9 mo	1100-1250	125-145
1 yr	1150-1300	120-135
2 yr	1350-1500	115-125
4 yr	1600-1800	100-110
6 yr	1800-2000	90-100
10 yr	2000-2500	70-85
14 yr	2200-2700	50-60
18 yr	2200-2700	40-50

From Behrman RE, Vaughan VC, editors: *Nelson textbook of pediatrics,* ed 13, Philadelphia, 1987, WB Saunders, p 115.

CALCULATION OF MAINTENANCE INTRAVENOUS FLUIDS FOR PEDIATRIC PATIENTS

1. Calculate weight of child in kilograms:

$$\text{Weight of child (in pounds)} \div \frac{2.2 \text{ lb}}{1 \text{ kg}} = \text{Weight in kilograms}$$

2. Allow 100 ml per kilogram for first 10 kg
3. Allow 50 ml per kilogram for second 10 kg
4. Allow 20 ml per kilogram for remainder of weight in kilograms
5. Divide total amount by 24 hours to obtain rate in milliliters per hour

ASSESSMENT OF URINARY OUTPUT

Urinary output should be 0.5 to 2 ml/kg/hr (depending on child's age and hydration status).

4 INTRAMUSCULAR INJECTIONS

Vastus Lateralis Site

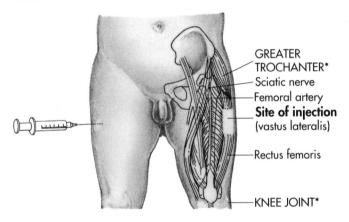

GREATER
TROCHANTER*
Sciatic nerve
Femoral artery
Site of injection
(vastus lateralis)

Rectus femoris

KNEE JOINT*

*Indicates locations of landmarks.

Ventrogluteal Site

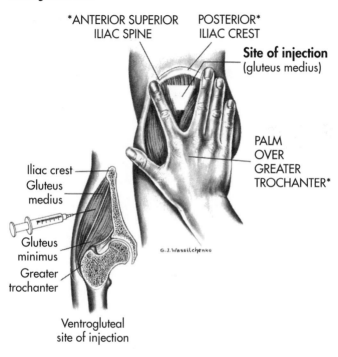

*ANTERIOR SUPERIOR ILIAC SPINE

POSTERIOR* ILIAC CREST

Site of injection
(gluteus medius)

PALM OVER GREATER TROCHANTER*

Iliac crest
Gluteus medius
Gluteus minimus
Greater trochanter

G.J. Wassilchenko

Ventrogluteal site of injection

---

*Indicates locations of landmarks.

Deltoid Site

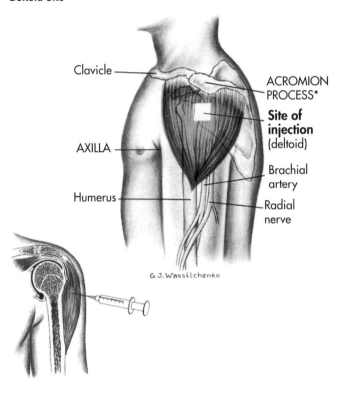

Clavicle

ACROMION
PROCESS*

**Site of
injection**
(deltoid)

AXILLA

Brachial
artery

Humerus

Radial
nerve

G.J.Wassilchenko

---

*Indicates locations of landmarks.

Dorsogluteal Site

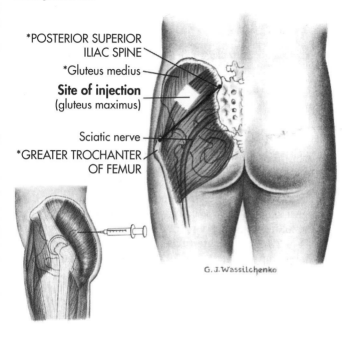

*POSTERIOR SUPERIOR
ILIAC SPINE

*Gluteus medius

Site of injection
(gluteus maximus)

Sciatic nerve

*GREATER TROCHANTER
OF FEMUR

G. J. Wassilchenko

*Indicates locations of landmarks.

5 EMERGENCY INFORMATION

RAPID CARDIOPULMONARY ASSESSMENT
Respiratory Assessment

A. Airway Patency
- Able to maintain independently
- Requires adjuncts/assistance to maintain

B. Breathing
Rate

Mechanics
  Retractions
  Grunting
  Accessory muscles
  Nasal flaring

Air entry
  Chest expansion
  Breath sounds
  Stridor
  Wheezing
  Paradoxical chest movement

Color

Cardiovascular Assessment
C. Circulation

Heart rate

Blood pressure
  Volume/strength of central pulses

Peripheral pulses
  Present/absent
  Volume/strength

Skin perfusion
  Capillary refill time*
  (consider ambient temperature)
  Temperature
  Color
  Mottling

CNS perfusion
  Responsiveness
    Awake
    Responds to voice
    Responds to pain
    Unresponsive
  Recognizes parents
  Muscle tone
  Pupil size
  Posturing

Modified from Chameides L, Hazinski MF, editors: *Textbook of pediatric advanced life support,* Dallas, 1994, American Heart Association.

*To measure capillary refill time (CRT), press the skin lightly on a central site, such as the forehead, or a peripheral site, such as the top of the hand, to produce a slight blanching. The time it takes for the blanched area to return to its original color is the capillary refill time. Capillary refill should be brisk (<2 seconds); prolonged CRT may be associated with poor systemic perfusion. Cool environmental temperature may also prolong CRT.

GUIDELINES FOR ENDOTRACHEAL TUBE AND SUCTION CATHETER SIZES*

Age	Internal diameter of tube (mm)	Suction catheter (French)
Term newborn	3.0-3.5†	6-8
6 mo	3.5-4.0†	8
18 mo	4.0-4.5†	8
3 yr	4.5-5.0†	8
5 yr	5.0-5.5†	10
6 yr	5.5†	10
8 yr	6.0‡	10
12 yr	6.5-7.0‡	10
16 yr	7.0-8.0‡	10
Adult female	7.5-8.0‡	12
Adult male	8.0-8.5‡	14

Modifed from Emergency Cardiac Care Committee and Subcommittees, American Heart Association: Guidelines for cardiopulmonary resuscitation and emergency cardiac care. VI. Pediatric advanced life support, *JAMA* 268(16):2262-2275, 1992; and Chameides L, Hazinski MF, editors: *Textbook of pediatric advanced life support,* Dallas, 1994, American Heart Association.

*Endotracheal tube selection for a child should be based on the child's size, not age. One size larger and one smaller should be allowed for individual variations.

†Uncuffed.

‡Cuffed.

CARDIAC ARREST DRUGS
*Drugs Used in Pediatric Advanced Life Support**

Drug	Dose	Remarks
Adenosine	0.1 to 0.2 mg/kg Maximum single dose: 12 mg	Rapid IV bolus
Atropine sulfate	0.02 mg/kg per dose	Minimum dose: 0.1 mg Maximum single dose: 0.5 mg in child, 1.0 mg in adolescent
Bretylium	5 mg/kg; may be increased to 10 mg/kg	Rapid IV
Calcium chloride 10%	20 mg/kg per dose	Give slowly
Dopamine hydrochloride	2-20 µg/kg per minute	α-Adrenergic action dominates at ≥15-20 µg/kg per minute
Dubtamine hydrochloride	2-20 µg/kg per minute	Titrate to desired effect
Epinephrine For bradycardia	IV/IO: 0.01 mg/kg (1:10,000) ET: 0.1 mg/kg (1:1000)	Be aware of effective dose of preservatives administered (if preservatives are present in epinephrine preparation) when high doses are used
For asystolic or pulseless arrest	First dose: IV/IO: 0.01 mg/kg (1:10,000) ET: 0.1 mg/kg (1:1000) Doses as high as 0.2 mg/kg may be effective Subsequent doses: IV/IO/ET: 0.1 mg/kg (1:1000) Doses as high as 0.2 mg/kg may be effective	Be aware of effective dose of preservatives administered (if preservatives are present in epinephrine preparation) when high doses are used

Modified from Chameides L, Hazinski MF, editors: *Textbook of pediatric advanced life support*, Dallas, 1994, American Heart Association.
*IV, Intravenous route; *IO,* intraosseous route; *ET,* endotracheal route.

Drugs Used in Pediatric Advanced Life Support—cont'd

Drug	Dose	Remarks
Epinephrine infusion	Initial at 0.1 µg/kg per minute Higher infusion dose used if asystole present	Titrate to desired effect (0.1-1.0 µg/kg per minute)
Lidocaine	1 mg/kg per dose	
Lidocaine infusion	20-50 µg/kg per minute	
Naloxone	If ≤ 5 years old or <20 kg: 0.1 mg/kg If >5 years old or >20 kg: 2.0 mg/kg	Titrate to desired effect
Sodium bicarbonate	1 mEq/kg per dose or 0.3 × kg × base deficit	Infuse slowly and only if ventilation is adequate

Preparation of Infusions

Drug	Preparation*	Dose
Epinephrine	0.6 × body weight (kg) equals milligrams added to diluent† to make 100 ml	Then 1ml/hr delivers 0.1 µg/kg per minute; titrate to effect
Dopamine, dobutamine	6 × body weight (kg) equals milligrams added to diluent to make 100 ml	Then 1 ml/hr delivers 1.0 µg/kg per minute; titrate to effect
Lidocaine	120 mg of 40-mg/ml solution added to 97 ml of 5% dextrose in water, yielding 1200 µg/ml solution	Then 1 ml/kg per hour delivers 20 µg/kg per minute

Modified from Chameides L, Hazinski MF, editors: *Textbook of pediatric advanced life support,* Dallas, 1994, American Heart Association.

*Standard concentration may be used to provide more dilute or more concentrated drug solution, but then individual dose must be calculated for each patient and each infusion rate:

$$\text{Infusion rate (ml/hr)} = \frac{\text{Weight (kg)} \times \text{Dose (µg/kg/min)} \times 60 \text{ min/hr}}{\text{Concentration (µg/ml)}}$$

†Diluent may be 5% dextrose in water, 5% dextrose in half-normal saline, normal saline, or Ringer's lactate.

FIRST AID FOR CHOKING*
Infant (Birth to 1 Year)
Conscious Infant
1. When obstruction by a foreign object is strongly suspected but the infant can cry, cough, or breathe, do not interfere.
2. If the infant cannot cry, cough, or breathe, deliver up to 5 back blows.
3. If this does not remove the object, give up to 5 chest thrusts.
   Repeat back blows and chest thrusts until the foreign object is expelled or the infant becomes unconscious.

If the Infant Becomes Unconscious
1. Using tongue-jaw lift, open mouth. If foreign object is seen, take it out.
2. Open airway (head-tilt/chin-lift); perform mouth-to-mouth/nose rescue breathing.
3. If unsuccessful, deliver up to 5 back blows followed by up to 5 chest thrusts.
4. If still unsuccessful, repeat sequence of tongue-jaw lift, rescue breathing, back blows, chest thrusts.

Child 1 to 8 Years
Conscious Child
1. Ask the child, "Are you choking?" If the child can speak, cough, or breathe, do not interfere.
2. If the victim cannot speak, cough, or breathe, or the cough is ineffective, perform abdominal thrusts (Heimlich maneuver) until the foreign body is expelled or until the child becomes unconscious.

Data from Chandra NC, Hazinski MF, editors: *Textbook of basic life support for healthcare providers,* Dallas, 1994, American Heart Association.
*These guidelines should not be used as substitutes for basic life support (BLS) training.

If the Child Becomes Unconscious

1. Using tongue-jaw lift, open mouth. If a foreign body is seen, take it out.
2. Open airway (head-tilt/chin-lift); perform mouth-to-mouth rescue breathing.
3. If unsuccessful, reposition head and try to ventilate again; if still obstructed, apply up to 5 abdominal thrusts.
4. If still unsuccessful, repeat sequence: abdominal thrusts, foreign body check, open airway, attempt rescue breathing.

Child Over 8 Years
Conscious Victim

1. Ask the victim: "Are you choking?" If the victim can speak, cough, or breathe, do not interfere.
2. If the victim cannot speak, cough, or breathe, or if the cough is ineffective, perform abdominal thrusts (Heimlich maneuver) until the foreign body is expelled or until the victim becomes unconscious.

If the Victim Becomes Unconscious

1. Using tongue-jaw lift, open mouth and perform finger sweep.
2. Open airway (head-tilt/chin-lift); perform mouth-to-mouth rescue breathing.
3. If unsuccessful, reposition head and try to ventilate again; if still obstructed, apply up to 5 abdominal thrusts.
4. If still unsuccessful, repeat sequence: abdominal thrusts, finger sweeps, open airway, attempt rescue breathing.

Be Persistent

Activate Emergency Medical Services (EMS) as soon as possible. Continue uninterrupted until advanced life support is available.

CALL-FOR-HELP NUMBER: 911 (or other emergency number).

CARDIOPULMONARY RESUSCITATION (CPR)*

Infant (Birth to 1 Year)

Place victim flat on his/her back on a hard surface and call for help.

1. If unconscious, open airway using head-tilt/chin-lift, or jaw-thrust maneuver if neck injury suspected.

   Look, listen, and feel for breathing for 5 seconds.

2. If not breathing, give 2 slow breaths (1 to 1½ seconds per breath). If airway is blocked, reposition head and try to give breaths. If still blocked, follow choking guidelines on p. 62.

3. Check brachial pulse.

   If pulse is present, give 1 breath every 3 seconds.

4. If there is no pulse, begin chest compressions.

   Depress sternum ½ to 1 inch. Perform 5 compressions to every 1 breath.

   After about 1 minute, recheck for a pulse and activate Emergency Medical Services (EMS).

Child 1 to 8 Years

Place victim on his/her back on a hard surface and call for help.

1. If unconscious, open airway (head tilt/chin-lift or jaw-thrust).

   Look, listen, and feel for breathing for 5 seconds.

2. If not breathing, begin rescue breathing. Give 2 rescue breaths (1 to 1½ seconds per breath). If airway is blocked, reposition head and try again to give breaths. If still blocked, follow choking guidelines on pp. 62-63.

3. Check carotid pulse.

   If pulse is present, give 1 rescue breath every 3 seconds.

Data from Chandra NC, Hazinski MF, editors: *Textbook of basic life support for healthcare providers,* Dallas, 1994, American Heart Association.

*These guidelines should not be used as substitutes for basic life support (BLS) training.

4. If there is no pulse, begin chest compressions.

   Depress sternum 1 to 1½ inches. Perform 5 compressions to every 1 breath.

   After about 1 minute, recheck for a pulse and activate EMS.

Child Over 8 Years

Place victim flat on his/her back on a hard surface and activate EMS.

1. If unconscious, open airway (head-lift/chin-lift or jaw thrust). Look, listen, and feel for breathing for 5 seconds.

2. If not breathing, begin rescue breathing. Give 2 slow breaths (1½ to 2 seconds per breath). If airway is blocked, reposition head and try again to give breaths. If still blocked, follow choking guidelines on p. 63.

3. Check carotid pulse.

   If pulse is present, give 1 breath every 5 seconds.

4. If there is no pulse, begin chest compressions.

   Depress sternum 1½ to 2 inches. Perform 15 compressions (rate: 80 to 100 per minute) to every 2 full breaths.

   At the end of 4 cycles, recheck for a pulse.

All Ages

If victim is breathing or resumes effective breathing, place in recovery position: (1) move head, shoulders, and torso simultaneously; (2) turn onto side; (3) leg not in contact with ground may be bent and knee moved forward to stabilize victim; (4) victim should not be moved in any way if trauma is suspected (unless in danger of further injury) and should not be placed in recovery position if rescue breathing or CPR is required.

APPROXIMATE WEIGHT PER AGE

Age	Weight (kg)
Newborn	5
6 mo	7
1 yr	10
2-3 yr	12-14
4-5 yr	16-18
6-8 yr	20-26
8-10 yr	26-32
10-14 yr	32-50
14 yr	50

1 kg = 2.2 lb.

6 COMMON LABORATORY TESTS

Test/specimen	Age/sex/reference	Conventional units	International units (SI)*
		Normal ranges	
Acetaminophen			
Serum or plasma	Therap. conc.	10-30 µg/ml	66-200 µmol/L
	Toxic conc.	>200 µg/ml	>1300 µmol/L
Ammonia nitrogen			
Plasma or serum	Newborn	90-150 µg/dl	64-107 µmol/L
	0-2 wk	79-129 µg/dl	56-92 µmol/L
	>1 mo	29-70 µg/dl	21-50 µmol/L
	Thereafter	15-45 µg/dl	11-32 µmol/L
Urine, 24 hr		500-1200 mg/d	36-86 mmol/d
Base excess			
Whole blood	Newborn	(−10)-(−2) mmol/L	(−10)-(−2) mmol/L
	Infant	(−7)-(−1) mmol/L	(−7)-(−1) mmol/L
	Child	(−4)-(+2) mmol/L	(−4)-(+2) mmol/L
	Thereafter	(−3)-(+3) mmol/L	(−3)-(+3) mmol/L

Modified from Behrman RE and others, editors: *Nelson textbook of pediatrics,* ed 15, Philadelphia, 1996, WB Saunders.

*Systeme International a'Unités.

Continued

Test/specimen	Age/sex/reference	Conventional units		International units (SI)*	
		Normal ranges			
		Premature (mg/dl)	Full term (mg/dl)	Premature (µmol/L)	Full term (µmol/L)
Bicarbonate (HCO₃)					
Serum	Arterial	21-28 mmol/L		21-28 mmol/L	
	Venous	22-29 mmol/L		22-29 mmol/L	
Bilirubin, total					
Serum	Cord	<2.0	<2.0	<34	<34
	0.1 d	8.0	<6.0	<137	<103
	1-2 d	12.0	<8.0	<205	<137
	2-5 d	16.0	<12.0	<274	<205
	Thereafter	2.0	0.2-1.0	<34	3.4-17.1
Bilirubin, direct (conjugated)					
Serum		0-0.2 mg/dl		0-3.4 µmol/L	
Bleeding time					
Blood from skin puncture					
Ivy	Normal	2-7 min		2-7 min	
	Borderline	7-11 min		7-11 min	
Simplate (G-D)		2.75-8 min		2.75-8 min	
C-reactive protein (CRP)					
Serum	Cord	52-1330 ng/ml		52-1330 µg/L	
	2-12 yr	67-1800 ng/ml		67-1800 µg/L	

Calcium, ionized			
Serum, plasma, or whole blood	Cord	5.0-6.0 mg/dl	1.25-1.50 mmol/L
	Newborn, 3-24 hr	4.3-5.1 mg/dl	1.07-1.27 mmol/L
	24-48 hr	4.0-4.7 mg/dl	1.00-1.17 mmol/L
	Thereafter	4.8-4.92 mg/dl	1.12-1.23 mmol/L
Calcium, total			
Serum	Cord	9.0-11.5 mg/dl	2.25-2.88 mmol/L
	Newborn, 3-24 hr	9.0-10.6 mg/dl	2.3-2.65 mmol/L
	24-48 hr	7.0-12.0 mg/dl	1.75-3.0 mmol/L
	4-7 d	9.0-10.9 mg/dl	2.25-2.73 mmol/L
	Child	8.8-10.8 mg/dl	2.2-2.70 mmol/L
	Thereafter	8.4-10.2 mg/dl	2.1-2.55 mmol/L
Carbon dioxide, partial pressure Pco_2			
Whole blood, arterial	Newborn	27-40 mm Hg	3.6-5.3 kPa
	Infant	27-41 mm Hg	3.6-5.5 kPa
	Thereafter: Male	35-48 mm Hg	4.7-6.4 kPa
	Female	32-45 mm Hg	4.3-6.0 kPa
Carbon dioxide, total (tCO_2)			
Serum or plasma	Cord	14-22 mEq/L	14-22 mmol/L
	Premature (1 wk)	14-27 mEq/L	14-27 mmol/L
	Newborn	13-22 mEq/L	13-22 mmol/L
	Infant, child	20-28 mEq/L	20-28 mmol/L
	Thereafter	23-30 mEq/L	23-30 mmol/L

*Systeme International a'Unités.

Continued

Test/specimen	Age/sex/reference	Conventional units			International units (SI)*		
		Normal ranges					
Cerebrospinal fluid (CSF)							
Pressure		70-180 mm water			70-180 mm water		
Volume	Child	60-100 ml			0.06-0.10 L		
	Adult	100-160 ml			0.10-0.16 L		
Chloride							
Serum or plasma	Cord	96-104 mmol/L			96-104 mmol/L		
(For sweat, see sodium.)	Newborn	97-110 mmol/L			97-110 mmol/L		
	Thereafter	98-106 mmol/L			98-106 mmol/L		
Cholesterol, total	1-3 yr	45-182 mg/dl			1.15-4.70 mmol/L		
	4-6 yr	109-189 mg/dl			2.80-4.80 mmol/L		
		Percentiles			*Percentiles*		
		5	**75**	**95**	**5**	**75**	**95**
	Male:						
	6-9 yr	126	172	191 mg/dL	3.26	4.45	4.94 mmol/L
	10-14 yr	130	179	204 mg/dL	3.36	4.63	5.28 mmol/L
	15-19 yr	114	167	198 mg/dL	2.95	4.32	5.12 mmol/L

		Percentiles			Percentiles		
		5	**75**	**95**	**5**	**75**	**95**
Female:	6-9 yr	122	173	209 mg/dL	3.16	4.47	5.41 mmol/L
	10-14 yr	124	174	217 mg/dL	3.21	4.50	5.61 mmol/L
	15-19 yr	125	175	212 mg/dL	3.23	4.53	5.48 mmol/L
Clotting time (Lee–White)							
Whole blood		5-8 min (glass tubes)			5-8 min		
		5-15 min (room temp)			5-15 min		
		30 min (silicone tube)			30 min		
Creatinine							
Serum	Cord	0.6-1.2 mg/dl			53-106 μmol/L		
	Newborn	0.3-1.0 mg/dl			27-88 μmol/L		
	Infant	0.2-0.4 mg/dl			18-35 μmol/L		
	Child	0.3-0.7 mg/dl			27-62 μmol/L		
	Adolescent	0.5-1.0 mg/dl			44-88 μmol/L		
	Adult: Male	0.6-1.2 mg/dl			53-106 μmol/L		
	Female	0.5-1.1 mg/dl			44-97 μmol/L		
Urine, 24 hr	Premature	8.1-15.0 mg/kg/24 hr			72-133 μmol/kg/24 hr		
	Full term	10.4-19.7 mg/kg/24 hr			92-174 μmol/kg/24 hr		
	1.5-7 yr	10-15 mg/kg/24 hr			88-133 μmol/kg/24 hr		
	7-15 yr	5.2-41 mg/kg/24 hr			46-362 μmol/kg/24 hr		

Continued

Systeme International a'Unités.

Test/specimen	Age/sex/reference	Conventional units	International units (SI)*
		Normal ranges	
Creatinine clearance (endogenous)			
Serum or plasma and urine	Newborn	40-65 ml/min/1.73 m²	
	<40 yr: Male	97-137 ml/min/1.73 m²	
	Female	88-128 ml/min/1.73 m²	
Digoxin			
Serum, plasma; collect at least 12 hr after dose	Therap. conc.		
	CHF	0.8-1.5 ng/ml	1.0-1.9 nmol/L
	Arrhythmias	1.5-2.0 ng/ml	1.9-2.6 nmol/L
	Toxic conc.		
	Child	>2.5 ng/ml	>3.2 nmol/L
	Adult	>3.0 ng/ml	>3.8 nmol/L
Erythrocyte (RBC) count			
Whole blood	Birth	4.0-6.6 million/mm³	4.0-6.6 × 10¹² cells/L
	3-6 mo	3.1-4.5 million/mm³	3.1-4.5 × 10¹² cells/L
	0.5-2 yr	4.0-6.6 million/mm³	4.0-6.6 × 10¹² cells/L
	2-6 yr	3.9-5.3 million/mm³	3.9-5.3 × 10¹² cells/L
	6-12 yr	4.0-5.2 million/mm³	4.0-5.2 × 10¹² cells/L
	12-18 yr: Male	4.5-5.3 million/mm³	4.5-5.3 × 10¹² cells/L
	Female	4.1-5.1 million/mm³	4.1-5.1 × 10¹² cells/L

Erythrocyte sedimentation rate (ESR)			
Whole blood			
Westergren (modified)	Child	0-10 mm/hr	0-10 mm/hr
	<50 yr: Male	0-15 mm/hr	0-15 mm/hr
	Female	0-20 mm/hr	0-20 mm/hr
Wintrobe	Child	0-13 mm/hr	0-13 mm/hr
	Adult: Male	0-9 mm/hr	0-9 mm/hr
	Female	0-20 mm/hr	0-20 mm/hr
Fibrinogen			
Plasma	Newborn	125-300 mg/dl	1.25-3.00 g/L
	Thereafter	200-400 mg/dl	2.00-4.00 g/L
Glucose†			
Serum	Newborn, 1 d	40-60 mg/dl	2.2-3.3 mmol/L
	Newborn, >1 d	50-90 mg/dl	2.8-5.0 mmol/L
	Child	60-100 mg/dl	3.3-5.5 mmol/L
	Thereafter	70-105 mg/dl	3.9-5.8 mmol/L
Whole blood	Adult	65-95 mg/dl	3.6-5.3 mmol/L
CSF	Adult	40-70 mg/dl	2.2-3.9 mmol/L
Urine (quantitative)		<0.5 g/d	<2.8 mmol/d
(qualitative)		Negative	Negative

*Systeme International a'Unités.
†Values for newborn vary according to different authorities.

Continued

		Conventional units	International units (SI)*
Test/specimen	**Age/sex/reference**	**Normal ranges**	
Hematocrit (HCT, Hct)			
Whole blood	1 d (cap)	48%-69%	0.48-0.69 vol. fraction
	2 mo	28%-42%	0.28-0.42 vol. fraction
	6-12 yr	35%-45%	0.35-0.45 vol. fraction
	12-18 yr: Male	37%-49%	0.37-0.49 vol. fraction
	Female	36%-46%	0.36-0.46 vol. fraction
Hemoglobin (Hb)			
Whole blood	1-3 d (cap)	14.5-22.5 g/dl	2.25-3.49 mmol/L
	2 mo	9.0-14.0 g/dl	1.40-2.17 mmol/L
	6-12 yr	11.5-15.5 g/dl	1.78-2.40 mmol/L
	12-18 yr: Male	13.0-16.0 g/dl	2.02-2.48 mmol/L
	Female	12.0-16.0 g/dl	1.86-2.48 mmol/L
Iron			
Serum	Newborn	100-250 µg/dl	17.90-44.75 µmol/L
	Infant	40-100 µg/dl	7.16-17.90 µmol/L
	Child	50-120 µg/dl	8.95-21.48 µmol/L
	Thereafter: Male	50-160 µg/dl	8.95-28.64 µmol/L
	Female	40-150 µg/dl	7.16-26.85 µmol/L
	Intoxicated child	280-2550 µg/dl	50.12-456.5 µmol/L
	Fatally poisoned child	>1800 µg/dl	>322.2 µmol/L

Iron-binding capacity, total (TIBC)			
Serum	Infant	100-400 µg/dl	17.90-71.60 µmol/L
	Thereafter	250-400 µg/dl	44.75-71.60 µmol/L
Lead			
Whole blood		<10 µg/dl	<0.48 µmol/L
Urine, 24 hr		<80 µg/L	<0.39 µmol/L
Leukocyte count (WBC count)		**× 1000 cells/mm³ (µl)**	**× 10⁹ cells/L**
Whole blood	Birth	9.0-30.0	9.0-30.0
	1-3 yr	6.0-17.5	6.0-17.5
	4-7 yr	5.5-15.5	5.5-15.5
	8-13 yr	4.5-13.5	4.5-13.5
	Adult	4.5-11.0	4.5-11.0
		× 1000 cells/mm³ (µl)	**× 10⁹ cells/L**
CSF	Premature	0-25 mononuclear	0-25
		0-100 polymorphonuclear	1-100
		0-1000 RBC	0-1000
	Newborn	0-20 mononuclear	0-20
		0-70 polymorphonuclear	0-70
		0-800 RBC	0-800
	Neonate	0-5 mononuclear	0-5
		0-25 polymorphonuclear	0-25
		0-50 RBC	0-50
	Thereafter	0-5 mononuclear	0-5

Systeme International a'Unités.

Continued

Test/specimen	Age/sex/reference	Conventional units	International units (SI)*
		Normal ranges	
Leukocyte differential count			
Whole blood	Myelocytes	0%	Number fraction 0
	Neutrophils—"bands"	3%–5%	Number fraction 0.03–0.05
		150-400 cells/mm³ (μl)	
	Neutrophils—"segs"	54%–62%	Number fraction 0.54–0.62
		3000-5800 cells/mm³ (μl)	
	Lymphocytes	25%–33%	Number fraction 0.25–0.33
		1500-3000 cells/mm³ (μl)	
	Monocytes	3%–7%	Number fraction 0.03–0.07
		285-500 cells/mm³ (μl)	
	Eosinophils	1%–3%	Number fraction 0.01–0.03
		50-250 cells/mm³ (μl)	
	Basophils	0%–0.75%	Number fraction 0-0.0075
		15-50 cells/mm³ (μl)	

Mean corpuscular hemoglobin (MCH)			
Whole blood	Birth	31-37 pg/cell	0.48-0.57 fmol/L
	3-6 mo	25-35 pg/cell	0.39-0.54 fmol/L
	0.5-2 yr	23-31 pg/cell	0.36-0.48 fmol/L
	2-6 yr	24-30 pg/cell	0.37-0.47 fmol/L
	6-12 yr	25-33 pg/cell	0.39-0.51 fmol/L
	12-18 yr	25-35 pg/cell	0.39-0.54 fmol/L
	18-49 yr	26-34 pg/cell	0.40-0.53 fmol/L
Mean corpuscular hemoglobin concentration (MCHC)			
Whole blood	Birth	30%-36% Hb/cell or g Hb/dl RBC	4.65-5.58 mmol or Hb/L RBC
	3 mo-2 yr	30%-36% Hb/cell or g Hb/dl RBC	4.65-5.58 mmol or Hb/L RBC
	2-18 yr	31%-37% Hb/cell or g Hb/dl RBC	4.81-5.74 mmol or Hb/L RBC
	>18 yr	31%-37% Hb/cell or g Hb/dl RBC	4.81-5.74 mmol or Hb/L RBC

*Systeme International a'Unités.

Continued

Test/specimen	Age/sex/reference	Conventional units	International units (SI)*
		Normal ranges	
Mean corpuscular volume (MCV)			
Whole blood	1-3 d (cap)	95-121 μm³	95-121 fl
	0.5-2 yr	70-86 μm³	70-86 fl
	6-12 yr	77-95 μm³	77-95 fl
	12-18 yr: Male	78-98 μm³	78-98 fl
	Female	78-102 μm³	78-102 fl
Osmolality			
Serum	Child, adult:	275-295 mOsmol/kg H₂O	
Urine, random		50-1400 mOsmol/kg H₂O, depending on fluid intake; after 12 hr fluid restriction: >850 mOsmol/kg H₂O	
Urine, 24 hr		≈300-900 mOsmol/kg H₂O	
Oxygen, partial pressure (Po₂)			
Whole blood, arterial	Birth	8-24 mm Hg	1.1-3.2 kPa
	5-10 min	33-75 mm Hg	4.4-10.0 kPa
	30 min	31-85 mm Hg	4.1-11.3 kPa
	>1 hr	55-80 mm Hg	7.3-10.6 kPa
	1 d	54-95 mm Hg	7.2-12.6 kPa
	Thereafter (decreases with age)	83-108 mm Hg	11-14.4 kPa

Test		Conventional	SI
Oxygen saturation (SaO$_2$)			
Whole blood, arterial	Newborn	85%-90%	Fraction saturated 0.85-0.90
	Thereafter	95%-99%	Fraction saturated 0.95-0.99
Partial thromboplastin time (PTT)			
Whole blood (Na citrate)			
Nonactivated		60-85 s (Platelin)	60-85 s
Activated		25-35 s (differs with method)	25-35 s
pH			
Whole blood, arterial	Birth, full term	7.11-7.36	43-77 nmol/L
	1 d	7.29-7.45	35-51 nmol/L
	Thereafter	7.35-7.45	35-44 nmol/L
Urine, random	Newborn/neonate	5-7	0.1-10 μmol/L
	Thereafter	4.5-8	0.01-32 μmol/L (average ≈1.0 μmol/L)
		(average ≈6)	
Platelet count (thrombocyte count)			
Whole blood (EDTA)	Newborn	84-478 × 10^3/mm^3 (μl)	84-478 × 10^9/L
	After 1 wk	150-400 × 10^3/mm^3 (μl)	150-400 × 10^9/L

*Systeme International a'Unités.

Continued

Test/specimen	Age/sex/reference	Conventional units	International units (SI)*
		Normal ranges	
Potassium			
Serum	Newborn	3.0-6.0 mmol/L	3.0-6.0 mmol/L
	Thereafter	3.5-5.0 mmol/L	3.5-5.0 mmol/L
Protein			
Serum, total	Newborn	4.6-7.4 g/dl	46-74 g/L
	1-7 yr	6.1-7.9 g/dl	61-79 g/L
	8-12 yr	6.4-8.1 g/dl	64-81 g/L
	13-19 yr	6.6-8.2 g/dl	66-82 g/L
Total			
Urine, 24 hr		1-14 mg/dl	10-140 mg/L
		50-80 mg/d (at rest)	50-80 mg/d
		<250 mg/d (after intense exercise)	<250 mg/d (after exercise)
Total			
CSF		Lumbar: 8-32 mg/dl	80-320 mg/L
Prothrombin time (PT)			
One-stage (Quick)	In general	11-15 sec (varies with type of thromboplastin)	11-15 sec
Whole blood (Na citrate)			
Two-stage modified (Ware and Seegers)	Newborn	Prolonged by 2-3 sec	Prolonged by 2-3 sec
Whole blood (Na citrate)		18-22 sec	18-22 sec

RBC count (See erythrocyte count.)			
Reticulocyte count			
Whole blood	Normal	0.5%-1.5% of erythrocytes or 25,000-75,000/mm³ (µl)	0.005-0.015 (number fraction) 25,000-75,000 × 10⁶/L
Salicylates			
Serum, plasma	Therap. conc.	15-30 mg/dl	1.1-2.2 mmol/L
	Toxic conc.	>30 mg/dl	>2.2 mmol/L
Sedimentation rate (See erythrocyte sedimentation rate.)			
Sodium			
Serum or plasma	Newborn	134-146 mmol/L	134-146 mmol/L
	Infant	139-146 mmol/L	139-146 mmol/L
	Child	138-145 mmol/L	138-145 mmol/L
	Thereafter	136-146 mmol/L	136-146 mmol/L
Sweat	Normal	<40 mmol/L	<40 mmol/L
	Indeterminate	45-60 mmol/L	45-60 mmol/L
	Cystic fibrosis	>60 mmol/L	>60 mmol/L

*Systeme International a' Unités.

Continued

Test/specimen	Age/sex/reference	Conventional units	International units (SI)*
		Normal ranges	
Specific gravity			
Urine, random	Adult	1.002-1.030	1.002-1.030
	After 12 hr fluid restriction	>1.025	>1.025
Urine, 24 hr		1.015-1.025	
Theophylline			
Serum, plasma	Therap. conc.		
	Bronchodilator	10-20 µg/ml	56-110 µmol/L
	Premature apnea	6-10 µg/ml	28-56 µmol/L
	Toxic conc.	>20 µg/ml	>166 µmol/L
Thrombin time			
Whole blood (Na citrate)		Control time ± 2 sec when control is 9-13 sec	Control time ± 2 sec when control is 9-13 sec

Triglycerides (TG)

Serum, after ≥12 hr fast

		mg/dl		g/L	
		M	F	M	F
	Cord blood	10-98	10-98	0.10-0.98	0.10-0.98
	0-5 yr	30-86	32-99	0.30-0.86	0.32-0.99
	6-11 yr	31-108	35-114	0.31-1.08	0.35-1.14
	12-15 yr	36-138	41-138	0.36-1.38	0.41-1.38
	16-19 yr	40-163	40-128	0.40-1.63	0.40-1.28
	20-29 yr	44-185	40-128	0.44-1.85	0.40-1.28

Urea nitrogen

Serum or plasma	Newborn	3-12 mg/dl	1.1-4.3 mmol urea/L
	Infant/child	5-18 mg/dl	1.8-6.4 mmol urea/L
	Thereafter	7-18 mg/dl	2.5-6.4 mmol urea/L

Urine volume

Urine, 24 hr	Newborn	50-300 ml/d	0.050-0.300 L/d
	Infant	350-550 ml/d	0.350-0.550 L/d
	Child	500-1000 ml/d	0.500-1.000 L/d
	Adolescent	700-1400 ml/d	0.700-1.400 L/d
	Thereafter: Male	800-1800 ml/d	0.800-1.800 L/d
	Female	600-1600 ml/d varies with intake and other factors)	0.600-1.600 L/d

WBC (See leukocyte.)

*Systeme International a'Unités.

SQ arm or thigh

1½ larger or obese

7 RECOMMENDED SCHEDULE FOR IMMUNIZATION OF HEALTHY INFANTS AND CHILDREN

deltoid 2 IM   *1" 23-25 guage*

vastus lateralis

Recommended age	Immunization(s)*
Birth	HBV
1-2 mo	HBV
2 mo	DTaP, Hib, IPV, Rv
4 mo	DTaP, Hib, IPV, Rv
6 mo	DTaP, Hib, Rv
6-18 mo	HBV, IPV
12-15 mo	Hib, MMR – *SQ*
12-18 mo	Varicella – *SQ*
15-18 mo	DTaP
4-6 yr	DTaP, IPV, MMR
14-16 yr; repeat every 10 yr throughout life	Td

Modified from American Academy of Pediatrics, Committee on Infectious Diseases: Recommended childhood immunization schedule-United States, January-December 1999, *Pediatrics* 103(1):181-182 (inset), 1999.

*Vaccine abbreviations: *HBV,* hepatitis B virus vaccine; *DTaP,* diphtheria and tetanus toxoids and acellular pertussis vaccine; *Hib, Haemophilus influenzae* type b conjugate vaccines; *IPV,* inactivated poliovirus vaccine; *MMR,* live measles, mumps, and rubella viruses vaccine; *Rv,* rotavirus; *Td,* adult tetanus toxoid (full dose) and diphtheria toxoid (reduced dose) for children ≥7 years and adults.

8 SELECTED RESOURCES ON PAIN AND IMMUNIZATION

Acute pain management in infants, children and adolescents: operative and medical procedures. Book contains federal medical practice guidelines written by a panel of experts. Available at no charge from the Agency for Health Care Policy and Research (AHCPR) Publications, PO Box 8527, Silver Spring, MD 20907; (800) 358-9295; www.ahcpr.gov.

Principles of analgesic use in the treatment of acute pain and cancer pain, ed 4, 1999. Booklet describing consensus guidelines for treating pain. From American Pain Society (APS), 4700 W. Lake Dr., Glenview, IL 60025-1485; (847) 375-4715; fax (847) 375-6315; e-mail: info@ampainsoc.org: www.ampainsoc.org/; or from Purdue Frederick Company, 100 Connecticut Ave., Norwalk, CT 06850-3950; (800) 733-1333 or (203) 853-0123, ext. 7378 or 7314; www.partnersagainstpain.com.

Management of acute pain: a practical guide. Book describing effective pain management strategies. Available from the International Association for the Study of Pain (IASP), 909 NE 43rd St., Suite 306, Seattle, WA 98105-6020; (206) 547-6409; e-mail: IASP@locke.hs.washington.edu; www.halcyon.com/iasp.

Cancer Pain Relief and Palliative Care in Children (In English; French and Spanish in preparation.) World Health organization in conjunction with IASP. 1998, ISBN 92-4-154512-7, 76 pp, Sw.fr.18-. Order from: WHO Distribution and Sales, 1211 Geneva 27, Switzerland. Price in developing countries: Sw.fr.12.60. In the U.S.: $16.20 plus $5 shipping and handling: Order no. 1150459. WHO Publications Center USA, 49 Sheridan Ave., Albany, NY 12210, USA; (518) 436-9686; fax: (518) 436-7433; e-mail: QCORP@compuserve.com.

Joint Commission on Accreditation of Healthcare Organizations (JCAHO) has established pain assessment and management standards and a toll-free hotline at (800) 994-6610 to encourage patients, their families, caregivers, and others to share concerns regarding quality of care issues at accredited health care organizations. Complaints (may be anonymous) may be sent by e-mail to: complaint@jcaho.org; faxed to the office of Quality Monitoring at (630) 792-5636; or mailed to the Office of Quality Monitoring, Joint Commission, One Renaissance Blvd, Oakbrook Terrace, IL, 60181. The pain standards are available from www.jcaho.org/standard/pm_hap.html

Pain Resource Center. Serves as a clearinghouse to disseminate information and resources to improve the quality of pain management. From City of Hope National Medical Center, Pain Resource Center, 1500 East Duarte Road, Duarte, CA 91010; (626) 359-8111, ext. 3829; fax (626) 301-8941; e-mail: mayday_pain@smtplink.coh.org; Web site: http://mayday.coh.org.

Whaley and Wong's Pediatric Pain Assessment Management by Donna Wong, PhD, RN. Videotape focuses on process of QUESTT for pain assessment and Six Rights for pharmacologic pain relief. Available from Mosby, 11830 Westline Industrial Drive, St. Louis, MO 63146: (800) 426-4545; fax (800) 535-9935; www.mosby.com.

Wong-Baker FACES Pain Rating Scale Reference Manual describing development and research of the scale is available from the Pain Resource Center, City of Hope National Medical Center, 1500 East Duarte Road, Duarte, CA 91010; (626) 359-8111, ext. 3829; fax (626) 301-8941; e-mail: mayday_pain@smtplink.coh.org. To obtain permission to use the scale, contact: Julie Lawley, WB Saunders, The Curtis Center, Independence Square West, Philadelphia, PA 19106; (800) 523-1649, ext. 8302; fax (215) 238-8483; or www.mosby.com/WOW/. A compilation of many pain scales, including the FACES, is available free from Purdue Frederick Company, 100 Connecticut Ave., Norwalk, CT 06850-3950; (800) 733-1333 or (203) 853-0123, ext. 7378 or 7314; e-mail www.partnersagainstpain.com.

Wong-Baker FACES Pain Rating Scale Pins. Pins may be purchased with coding of 0-5 and 0-10 from Linda Toth, PO Box 2984, Sanford, NC 27331; phone (919) 498-1158; or fax (919) 498-3993.

Wong on Web. Internet access to numerous documents and other resource data compiled by Donna Wong. Web address: www.mosby.com/WOW/.

American Academy of Pediatrics (AAP) and the Centers for Disease Control and Prevention's (CDC) Advisory Committee on Immunization Practices (ACIP) are primary sources of information about immunization: American Academy of Pediatrics, 141 Northwest Point Boulevard, PO Box 747, Elk Grove Village, IL 60009-0747; phone (800) 433-9016; fax (847) 228-1281; e-mail www.aap.org; Centers for Disease Control and Prevention, 1600 Clifton Road, NE, Atlanta, GA 30333; phone: (404) 639-3311; information hotline, (800) 232-2522 or (800) 232-7468; international travel hotline, (877) 394-8747; Spanish hotline (800) 232-0233; e-mail: www.cdc.gov; or visit the National Immunization Program at CDC Web page, www.cdc.gov/nip/

Mortality and Morbidity Report (MMWR) contains comprehensive reviews of the literature as well as important background data regarding vaccine efficacy and side effects. To receive an electronic copy, send an e-mail message to listserv@listserv.cdc.gov. The body content should read: SUBscribe mmwr-toc. Electronic copy also is available from CDC's World Wide Web server at www.cdc.gov/ or from CDC's file transfer protocol server at ftp.cdc.gov. To subscribe for paper copy, contact Superintendent of Documents, U.S. Government Printing Office, Washington, DC 20402; phone (202) 512-1800.

Immunization Gateway: Your Vaccine Fact-Finder at www.immunofacts.com provides direct links to all the best vaccine resources on the Internet.

Vaccine Information Statements can be downloaded from the **Immunization Action Coalition's** Web site at www.immunize.org/vis/ or the CDC Web site at www.cdc.gov/nip/publications/vis/.

The **Whaley-Wong Update series** includes information on changes in immunization information: www.mosby.com/WOW/.

Conversion of Pounds to Kilograms for Pediatric Weight

Pounds → ↓	0	1	2	3	4
0	0.00	0.45	0.90	1.36	1.81
10	4.53	4.98	5.44	5.89	6.35
20	9.07	9.52	9.97	10.43	10.88
30	13.60	14.06	14.51	14.96	15.42
40	18.14	18.59	19.05	19.50	19.95
50	22.68	23.13	23.58	24.04	24.49
60	27.21	27.66	28.22	28.57	29.03
70	31.75	32.20	32.65	33.11	33.56
80	36.28	36.74	37.19	37.64	38.10
90	40.82	41.27	41.73	42.18	42.63
100	45.36	45.81	46.26	46.72	47.17
110	49.89	50.34	50.80	51.25	51.71
120	54.43	54.88	55.33	55.79	56.24
130	58.96	59.42	59.87	60.32	60.78
140	63.50	63.95	64.41	64.86	65.31
150	68.04	68.49	68.94	69.40	69.85
160	72.57	73.02	73.48	73.93	74.39
170	77.11	77.56	78.01	78.47	78.92
180	81.64	82.10	81.55	83.00	83.46
190	86.18	86.68	87.09	87.54	87.99
200	90.72	91.17	91.62	92.08	92.53